100 Years of Medicine

100 Years of Medicine

*Louis M. Soletsky, M.D., FACP with
David Soletsky, M.D.*

Writers Club Press
San Jose New York Lincoln Shanghai

100 Years of Medicine

Writers Club Press
an imprint of iUniverse, Inc.

For information address:
iUniverse, Inc.
5220 S. 16th St., Suite 200
Lincoln, NE 68512
www.iuniverse.com

ISBN: 0-595-22925-5

Printed in the United States of America

Contents

PREFACE

The germination of a book can be related to many factors, but in this particular book a singular factor is paramount. During the academic year of 1996, I had occasion to be involved in a teaching exercise with the first year medical residents at the Long Island Jewish Hospital. I was teamed with a psychiatrist, Dr. Jim Gordon, in a course called *Advanced Clinical Skills* (ACS). This course was an attempt to offer support and insight, as well as training, to young physicians as they had their first contacts with responsibility and illness combined. Most medical students have no responsibility when they see illnesses so, in effect, the first year of training in hospitals represents the first time that young doctors are faced with the responsibility for their own decisions in patient care. For many, this is very traumatic and the course was designed to alleviate some of the anxiety, as well as educate.

During several of these sessions, I had occasion to relate anecdotes from the practice of either my late father or myself. My father practiced medicine for 53 years in New York and I have practiced medicine for 47 years, hence the title of this book. Some of these anecdotes had a point, while others were merely interesting, but they were very well received in almost all cases by the young doctors, and by Dr. Gordon. At some point, Dr. Gordon said, "You should put these in a book." This effort represents the outcome of that germination.

ACKNOWLEDGMENTS

This book could not have been written without my father, who practiced medicine in New York for 53 years. During that entire time, he was a minute observer of the human foibles and the human condition and he delighted in sharing his insights with me from the days when I was quite a young child. Perhaps, it is a consequence of this that I have never had any desire other than to become a physician for a long as I can remember, and was utterly fortunate to have been able to do so.

This book could not have been produced without the skilled and devoted assistance of Mary Famulare and Victoria C. Soletsky.

HISTORY

David Soletsky was born on February 5, 1894, in the family apartment at 6 Allen Street delivered by a mid-wife. The building in question was an old world tenement, and had a privy in the backyard. He attended public school in New York City, graduated from the City College of New York and stayed to obtain a Master's degree in bacteriology. Incidentally, he was elected to Phi Beta Kappa. He attended Harvard Medical School from 1916 to 1920, and then spent one year as an intern and one year as a house physician at the Mount Sinai Hospital in New York before starting a private practice in the building where his family lived at 66 West 88th Street.

Louis M. Soletsky was born on March 4, 1927, delivered by his father in the father's private office, then at 38 Fort Washington Avenue in Manhattan. He attended New York City public schools, graduated from New York University in 1945, served one year on active duty in the United States Navy, and then attended the Hahnemann Medical College from 1946 to 1950. During that period he also was on weekend duty in the United States Naval Reserve, stationed on a submarine in the Philadelphia Navy Yard. During medical school he also clerked at the Philadelphia General Hospital, the Sacred Heart Hospital in Norristown, PA, the Women's Homeopathic Hospital in Philadelphia, and the Rockaway Beach Hospital in Queens, NY. Following graduation he was trained at the Jewish Memorial Hospital in New York City, Metropolitan Hospital on Welfare Island, Willard Parker Hospital, Queens General Hospital in Jamaica, NY, and the Boston City Hospital. He entered private practice at 81-52 Little Neck Parkway, Bellerose, NY.

THE FORK IN THE NECK

One evening during office hours, my father received an emergency call from a young woman who lived down the block, in an apartment with her husband. She insisted that he come over immediately because her husband was seriously injured. My father left the patients in the office and walked down the block with his medical bag, and into the apartment involved. The young woman ushered him into the kitchen where her husband was sitting rigidly at the kitchen table, clutching the edges of the table tightly with both hands. An ordinary dinner fork was sticking out of the side of his neck and a small amount of blood was trickling down. The fork was not deeply imbedded in the patient's neck and after assessing the situation, my father took a sterile gauze, cleaned the area a bit, pressed on the tissues involved, removed the fork and put a large dressing in place. He then asked the wife how this had happened. She pouted gently and said, "I threw it at him." My father said "You threw the fork at him?" "Oh, no," she said, "I threw the plate, the knife, the fork, the spoon, the glasses, the tea cup, everything on the table at him. But the fork stuck in his neck."

TETANUS

In 1951, as a young resident, I had occasion to admit a 13 year old with the acute spasms of frank clinical tetanus. Tetanus, or lockjaw, a disease that is hardly seen anymore, was much more common in the days before appropriate immunizations. Sadly, this young man had not been immunized, and somewhere along the way had scraped his knee on the street. In those days, there were still horses and there were appropriate droppings on the street, and horse manure is a very rich source of tetanus spores. Apparently, some got into the wound and managed to develop and produce the toxins that cause these hideous convulsive-like spasms. I researched the situation, obtained consultation with my attending, and we proceeded, after desensitizing the patient to horse serum, to give him enormous amounts of tetanus anti-toxin. We even injected the toxin all around and underneath the abrasion on his knee, which we assumed was the source of infection and then had the entire abrasion surgically removed. The patient was placed in a dark private room and nursed continually by the student nurses who were available to us. This all occurred, by the way, in the old Willard Parker Contagious Disease Hospital, long since closed. Various medications were used in an attempt to prevent the terrible spasms, none of them completely successful, and the days trickled by. Each morning as I came in, I first visited this patient, slipping silently into his room and examining him very gently. He continued to have periodic spasms. The medical textbooks at the time assured me that if the patient could be kept alive for 21 days, the spasms would disappear and the patient would recover. On the 21st morning, he was alive and my elation knew no bounds. He was still quite ill, but he was going to stop his spasms and get well. On the 22nd morning, he still had spasms, but he was here and the spasms were going to stop and he was going to get well. He died early in the morning on the 23rd day. To this day, the sense of despair that enveloped me then is fresh in my mind, and the name of this patient, which I will not record here, is indelibly imprinted in my memory. He was supposed to get well 47 years ago; I kept him alive the requisite 21 days, and he died anyway. Obviously medical science did not and sadly, does not have all the answers. As I write this, I can still feel the sense of impotence in the face of overwhelming medical disaster.

ADOPTION

Adoption has become an industry in our society. Adoptions were much simpler many years ago. I can remember vividly, since my father was very proud of it, a situation in which a young woman who was "in trouble" was admitted to the hospital and delivered a fine baby. The mother's thumbprint on the birth certificate somehow got smudged a little. The baby's foot however, was very neatly imprinted. The birth mother left through the back door of the hospital and my own father carried the baby, now three days old, down the steps in the front of the hospital and handed the baby through a car window to the baby's mother. Because, you see, that woman's name appeared on the hospital record as the mother. Considering all the circumstances, this may have been a wonderful trouble-free adoption since anybody searching the records afterward would find a useless thumbprint and a baby born to Mrs. So-and-so, who was the baby's mother. At the time, and I was a teenager, it seemed like a happy solution to me also. As time passed, I began to wonder what would have happened if the baby had been born with some terrible impairment. Fortunately, that did not occur, and I am sure this was not the only such "adoption" that my father arranged.

One of the other ways that out of wedlock births were disguised was to register the mother as her mother, in other words the grandmother would be having the baby on paper, to avoid problems later on. Obviously the grandmother who had children would have one more change of life baby and her daughter sent away for a few months to cooperative relatives would not have the stigma of an out of wedlock birth attached. The world has changed, of course, and nobody seems to be the least bit concerned anymore about out of wedlock births.

EUTHANASIA

In the course of this book I am sure that I will find many instances where there is room for a discussion of euthanasia. I have often felt that I didn't go to medical school to kill people, I went to medical school to help people. Unfortunately there are times when people cannot be cured and one has to wonder what the appropriate definition then of the word "help", in medical terms, might be. Years ago, my father had a bottle with 30 or 40 morphine hypodermic tablets. This is not the way morphine is distributed today, but in those days, the doctor carried morphine in a little vial of individual soluble tablets. The tablets were dissolved in a spoonful of water over an alcohol lamp, drawn up in a syringe, and then injected into the patient. The tablets would also dissolve very quickly in juice or soup, so it was not difficult to swallow a great many morphine tablets. At times when my father was dealing with patients who seemed to be suffering terribly, he would "forget" the bottle of morphine tablets in the sick room. The offer was never taken up and in fact every time he would quickly get a phone call saying, "Doctor, you forgot some medicine, we'll run it over to the office."

INFERTILITY

One of the complaints of patients, one that persists to this day, is the failure of a married couple to produce a baby. This can be extremely disturbing and I need not dwell upon how disturbing this is. Suffice to say that when my father was in practice only a few years (I would think this could never happen today), a young couple came to ask his help in getting the wife pregnant. As part of the history taking, my father inquired about sexual activity and sexual positions and this sort of thing. The young woman involved was rather chubby, with a rather large abdomen and a retracted belly button. After some care in listening and describing, my father ascertained that the couple involved was having intercourse using this orifice. It was of course not surprising in that case that they did not obtain a pregnancy. Oddly enough it did not seem so terribly surprising that they did not know any better. My father proceeded to instruct them in the proper location for obtaining sexual congress. Surprise! A pregnancy rather quickly ensued.

FAMILY

This little story concerns my cousin, Joe. Joe, my father's brother's son, as a six-year-old, poked an orange pit into his ear and neglected to mention it to anybody. The orange pit swelled up and his ear became quite painful. His father, who was also a physician, attempted to remove it, but the pain on just touching the orange pit was so severe that Joe would not allow removal. In addition, the orange pit's taper made it very difficult to get a grip on the pit to even try to remove it. The two brothers, both physicians of course, finally decided to attempt anesthesia for removal and I was invited to help out. I was nine or ten at the time and we worked in Joe's father's office, which was in the family home. The anesthetic decided upon was open drop ether and after a few minutes of lessons, I was given the job of doling out the ether once Joe had been put to sleep by my father. At that point, I continued an occasional drop of ether through the mask (an ordinary gauze mask, by the way) while my father and his brother attempted to get a grip on this tightly stuck, slippery orange pit. They finally took an ear instrument that had a small screw thread upon it, screwed it into the orange pit, and then with that plus a small forceps were able to dislodge the pit and remove it. As it came out, I was told to remove the ether mask and stop dripping the ether. I might mention that since my face was very near to my cousin Joe's face, I probably was pretty whimsical on the ether myself by that time. In a few minutes, Joe responded, woke up, vomited, which was the usual thing with ether, and as he was leaning over the vomit bowl (called by doctors an emesis basin or kidney basin) he looked around and said, "I hate everybody in this house." However, he didn't put any more orange pits in his ear.

DEATH

My father practiced medicine in New York City from 1920 to 1973 and in fact saw seven patients in his private office the night before he died. He died the following evening of a massive heart attack, not long before office hours were to begin. A few patients had to be turned away because he often worked by appointment, but the most poignant was in a telephone call. A gentleman called early during office hours begging to be allowed to come in that evening because he felt terrible. My father's secretary explained to him gently that the doctor had passed away that very night, and of course she could not offer him an appointment. The response on the telephone "My God, I knew I should've come in last night!"

CONFIDENTIALITY

Young physicians are constantly told that everything they learn from patients is confidential to be repeated to no one. This was a lesson that gets repeated frequently during medical school and it was one that we often reiterated during the ACS meetings at Long Island Jewish. Along the way, I told them a personal story. When I was a young physician, I attended a family wedding and there met a rather cute young woman whose mother was a good friend of my aunt's. I proceeded to start going out with her, which was of course no secret, since her mother and my mother and my aunt were all constantly talking to each other. Although not a word was said, I was very aware that my father was very unhappy with this relationship, although my mother seemed very happy about it. Nothing was ever said, but I got very strong vibes concerning this young woman. Nothing much came of it, and after a while we stopped seeing one another and I completely forgot about the matter. Years later, I had occasion to chat with my father about the issues of confidentiality and he had an anecdote to tell me. He said, "Do you remember that young woman you dated whose mother is a friend of your Aunt Anna's?" I said "Oh yes, I remember her, you didn't like it." He said, "It wasn't that I didn't like it. It was that I had treated that young woman, not once, but twice for gonorrhea." I must tell you that in those days when I was a young man, a young girl from a nice family who had gonorrhea twice was really a slut. Nonetheless, my father never said one word to me despite the fact that I felt his disapproval. I might mention, young doctors today who hear this story immediately equate this to the AIDS epidemic and find it very difficult to maintain confidentiality under such circumstances. Gonorrhea they feel was a curable treatable disease, while AIDS is hardly treatable or poorly treatable and apparently incurable. It's a difficult dichotomy for young physicians.

While I'm on the subject of weddings, I think of another family wedding I went to as a young physician where there was literally <u>one</u> nice looking single woman at the party. I was trying my new line, (I was an intern at the time) and as I danced with her I assured her that she could trust me because I was a doctor. I didn't get the feeling of an enormously positive reception, but one does the best one can. I happened to be dancing with my mother shortly afterward while the young woman was dancing with another young man. As we went by, I heard him say, "You can trust me, honey, I'm a rabbi." He took her home.

CHRISTIAN SCIENCE

During the years of his practice, my father treated several people who were Christian Science practitioners. Christian Science believes, of course, in the power of prayer to cure illnesses and it seemed a little odd that Christian Science practitioners would seek out the services of a physician. Nonetheless, they did and my father was quite pleased with the fact that they did. At the time, there was considerable disdain in the medical community about the powers of Christian Science and prayer. As we learn more about the immune system today and the fact that faith may well have an effect upon the immune system, perhaps prayer for some people at least in some circumstances has more power than we might first imagine.

While I'm on the subject of Christian Science, there is an anecdote that to this day distresses me greatly. I experienced this when I was a medical examiner, where I was sent to the home of man who had just died to make the appropriate medical decisions for the medical examiner's office. The man involved was in his forty's, a business executive, who while at work developed an excruciating pain in his great toe. His secretary, who was present at the death scene, told me that he complained only of this excruciating pain in his toe, but that he also turned gray and got terribly sweaty and just a little bit breathless. He looked so ill that she proceeded to get his automobile, bring it around to the door of his business and then drive him close to an hour to his home. All the way in the car, he continued to complain bitterly only of pain in the toe and he continued to look gray, sweaty and very ill. When he got to his home he went to bed and his wife called the Christian Science practitioner. The practitioner proceeded to pray for him and the patient continued to suffer excruciating pain in the toe for the next several hours before he died. Since I was the medical examiner, I decided that this case required an autopsy. Autopsy revealed a fresh clot in one of his main coronary arteries with a good-sized area of acutely damaged heart muscle. Examination of the toe showed nothing whatsoever that I could see that was abnormal. The fact that this poor man did not even obtain pain relief for his excruciating toe pain was bad enough, but the fact that he was not seen by a doctor to attempt to diagnose and treat his coronary condition was more distressing to me. Despite the power of faith, I have had difficulty accepting Christian Science as a viable form of medical care, but obviously everyone is entitled to their own religious beliefs.

POLICE

When I was a young doctor, the police were very helpful and one always found them cooperative in circumstances when a physician's situation was challenged. I was an intern, and occasionally made night calls for my father to allow him to sleep. I got a call one night through his answering service that the mother of a very famous columnist needed assistance. I went to the house to find a fascinating physical situation. This woman, an extremely obese woman, slept in a double bed in a very small bedroom. In fact, you entered the bedroom at the foot of the bed. There was a small aisle to walk along the foot of the bed and then a very tiny isle along one side of the bed and against that wall was a huge chest of drawers. This aisle at its best was perhaps two feet wide. Somehow this enormously fat lady had rolled into the crack between the bed and the wall, in the process had pushed the bed out from the wall until it was resting against the front of this huge chest of drawers, and could go no further. She was wedged in down on the floor, half underneath the bed and half in this narrow space that the bed had moved over from. She had an elderly housekeeper who lived with her, who had called me. This woman would not be any real assistance in getting the patient, dressed only in a nighty, back into bed. I called the police. Two squad cars with four jovial Irish policemen responded to me. I explained the situation, they grinned a little and we proceeded to maneuver this lady back into her bed. We did this by the five of us kneeling across her bed, reaching down into this crack where she was, getting a grip on something and the five of us on the count of three heaved her back up onto the bed. At this point, the obese lady totally exploded with laughter. She found the situation so utterly hilarious

14

and of course once she did, the five of us, and even the housekeeper began to laugh, too. We all thanked the policemen profusely, pushed the bed back solidly against the wall and asked her the next time she rolled out of bed would she please roll the other way rather than getting jammed in. She had trouble stopping her laughter, but nonetheless assured me it wouldn't happen again.

THE BEST LAID PLANS

Shortly after I went into practice, I was called to see an elderly woman in her early seventies, who had been moved into her son's home because she had become unable to handle her own affairs. I found her not particularly impaired mentally, but rather because of failing vision and hearing she really could no longer live alone. A decision was made by her son and daughter-in-law that they would add a room and bath on the back of their home for grandma to live in. They had three small children and the thought expressed to me by the daughter-in-law was that after the old lady passed on, this would be a lovely family and party room for the children while they were growing up. The years went by and I saw the woman mostly at home because of her physical impairments and she became a rather difficult and cantankerous house-guest and definitely a thorn in the daughter-in-law's side. Nonetheless, a decision had been made, caregivers were hired and the grandma continued to live in the room that was built for her. She lived to be ninety-seven years old, by which time all the children had grown and gone without ever having the new family room to use since grandma continued to live in it.

This unfortunate daughter-in-law seemed to specialize in episodes of bad judgment. She had a very large German shepherd dog, which was the family watchdog. Since she fed the dog and walked the dog, obviously the dog adored her and would protect her at all costs. The dog had one peculiarity—he hated the mailman. He would bark ferociously when the mailman appeared and if he was out, the mailman would not go anywhere near the house. In addition, every once in a while, he would mangle the mail. One day this woman was in a great hurry to go somewhere and she ran out the door, slammed it behind her and went to her car. As she went to get into her car, she realized she had both her keys and her husband's set of keys. Since he was still home, if she had taken his keys, he would have been stuck in the house. Consequently, she promptly ran back to her front door and pushed his set of keys through the mail slot. Unfortunately, she was wearing gloves. As she pushed the keys through the mail slot, her own beloved dog bit her on the hand, obviously not recognizing her gloved hand. She was furious, although not seriously injured, but she opened the door. The moment the dog saw her, he was so upset since he obviously realized what he'd done, that he let go of both bowel and bladder right in the front hall.

I might mention, I recall another anecdote that daughter-in-law told me in which she heard a loud boom in her basement and went down to find water pouring out of a burst pipe. She frantically looked for the valve to shut off the leak, could not find it and called her husband at work. She, by this time, was frantic as the water was truly pouring into her finished basement. Her husband, on the phone, said to her "Stop being so upset, you know where the shut off valve is." She screamed into the phone, "I can't remember. Tell me where it is!", and he of course said, "Calm down, you know where it is, you just have to think about it." Oddly enough that marriage did not end in divorce.

ANCIENT HISTORY

I have a volume that represents the clinical/pathological conferences at the Johns Hopkins Medical School and Hospital in 1912. It is a book that makes me feel very humble. It is clear that, for example, the awareness at Johns Hopkins, at least of the diagnosis, treatment and outcomes for lung cancer, was not really different than what we have today. That the diagnosis, treatment and outcomes for amputations related to gangrene and hardening of the arteries was not significantly different from what we have today. In fact, it is obvious that medicine has not come nearly as far as most doctors would like to think. Obviously, Johns Hopkins may well have been far superior to the average run-of-the-mill medical care in 1912, but the slopes in many areas of medicine become extremely obvious when reading this book.

THE OLD DAYS

Prior to World War II, the only real antibiotic available to physicians was sulfanilamide. This became available in the late 1930's, but when my father started practice in the 1920's, there were no antibiotics. In fact, he told me that in medical school he had been in a coma for three weeks with erysipelas and the doctors at Harvard Medical School, where he was a student, expected him to die. He survived however, without the need for antibiotics at that time. He also recalled vividly, and introduced me to, a very nice young woman who was quite deaf. In 1938, when she was twelve, she had been diagnosed with acute meningitis, an illness which, at that time, represented a death sentence. The rare patient with meningitis who survived was left with hideous brain damage, usually chronic convulsions, and had no quality of life to speak of. My father had just learned of this new drug called sulfanil-amide. He treated her with it and she survived. However, she did lose her hearing. At the time, quite frankly, despite the loss of hearing, her survival as a whole human being was seen as a true miracle and, as you can imagine, to a physician who had watched patients die of infections for years, the ability to treat infection effectively was close to magic.

TUBERCULOSIS

Many years ago, my father took care of a very nice Irish family, one of whose sons became a wonderful doctor, Dr. Lucas, but this story dates back to when Dr. Lucas and I were teenagers. His mother developed a cough and a little fever and some sweats at night. She ignored it as long as she could, but finally came to see my father. He examined her very carefully, pointed to the top of the left side of her chest and said, "You have a cavity there. It is almost certainly tuberculosis. You must go to the hospital." He arranged to get her admitted to the Presbyterian Hospital, an extremely fine hospital, of course, where she was on the teaching service. She was in the hospital for two weeks, had many tests, many visits and finally the day came when the professor made grand rounds. He swept into the ward, accompanied by some fifteen staff physicians, interns and residents. They crowded around her bed. He asked her to sit up in bed, he pointed to her chest and he said, "You have a tubercular cavity right there." She answered, "My doctor told me that in ten minutes in his office. Give me my clothes, I'm going home." And that's exactly what she did and, home in bed, she proceeded to control the disease and recover.

HOSPITALS

I

It may surprise both doctors and patients today, but fifty years ago, hospitals were constantly filled and it was extremely difficult to get patients into the hospital. In fact, it was so difficult that many groups of doctors would spend their own money to build a hospital so they would have beds for their patients. As you may imagine, when beds were tight, the doctors who owned the hospital, saw themselves as privileged characters with entree to the few remaining beds. I recall covering for a physician, who was away. Making a house call, I found one of his patients literally sitting up on the edge of his bed, vomiting blood into an ordinary bucket and there was close to an inch of his blood already in the bucket. I immediately went to the phone and called the hospital, where I was told that they were terribly sorry, but they did not have any beds. I should mention the doctor I was covering was an owner of the hospital. At that moment, the wife took the telephone out of my hand and said, "Just a moment, I don't think you understand. Dr. Soletsky is just covering Dr. So-and-so, this is Dr. So-and-so's patient." A bed immediately appeared. It seems that the patients understood the system better than I did.

II

I made a house call to one of my patients who had developed acute meningitis, an infection of the brain that I have previously mentioned. This is a definite emergency. I called all three of the hospitals where I worked at those times, and not one had a bed. I finally called the chief resident at the teaching hospital where I worked, and managed to get

21

the patient into one of his beds, a service bed, not available ordinarily for private patients. They made room since meningitis is an interesting disease. I should mention that nobody in their right mind should ever have what young doctors consider an "interesting disease". These are either the most disfiguring, the most hideous, the most acute, the most unpleasant or in some way, the most awful or unusual illnesses to have which, of course, makes them the most "interesting" illnesses to young physicians.

III

Hospitals have changed a lot. I'm sure that's not a statement that everyone does not realize, but hospitals have changed for so many reasons that it is difficult to even know where to begin. Perhaps a good illustration will be what I call "the 21-day coronary". In the original days, the Blue Cross Hospital Insurance Policy covered a patient for 21 days of semi-private care. A coronary artery occlusion, or a heart attack in simple parlance, was certainly a serious illness and almost every patient admitted with that diagnosis went home from the hospital on the 22nd morning. Today, patients with such illnesses may go home the next day, three days later, or 5 or 10 days later, but it is only the most unusual case that stays much over a week and only the hideously complicated cases would be in the hospital 21 days. This is only a small indication of the changes.

IV

When my father was an intern, Mt. Sinai Hospital had a loud paging system to summon its doctors, but of course no beepers. Frequently, the physicians would be called to a distant floor and would run for the elevator. In those days, the elevators were operated by people, usually men, and somehow friction developed between the house staff and the elevator operators. A doctor would be running to answer a page and he would frantically try to signal the elevator operator to wait for him and the operators began slamming their doors and taking off. As you can imagine, everybody involved became angrier and angrier until finally a notice appeared on the doctor's bulletin board. It read, "Please be polite to our elevator operators! We have no trouble recruiting doctors."

V

While I was a resident at the Boston City Hospital my father drove up from New York to visit me. I promptly took him to my room since I had a rather nice private room on the top floor of a four-story building, which appeared to contain no patients other than a small wing used as a student nurse infirmary. Since I was on the top floor I looked out on trees and had a pretty good breeze most of the time, and I was quite proud of my digs. My father walked into my room and burst out laughing. I saw nothing particularly funny about this and quizzed him on what was so funny in my room and he said, "When I was a medical student this was the main Boston City Hospital's hospital building and I treated patients regularly in this room." I said to him, "But surely they had wards." He said, "No, the original hospital building had small rooms." And it was actually quite a small hospital when he was a medical student.

When I arrived at the Boston City Hospital as a resident in June of 1953, the hospital was still abuzz about a disaster in the Coconut Grove nightclub, the infamous Thanksgiving nightclub fire. This nightclub fire had involved hundreds of casualties in a disastrous fire in which the people trying to get out the door jammed a revolving door so that nobody could get out and, consequently, many, many people were injured. The night and early morning of the fire, I was told, Massachusetts General Hospital took six patients, New England Deaconess Hospital took four patients, Peter Bent Brigham Hospital took six patients, and over 200 patients were sent to Boston City Hospital. They mobilized their house staff and, in effect, gave each house staffer one patient. This meant even dermatology and physical therapy residents and all the interns were handed an injured patient. The operating rooms worked 36 hours straight and the hospital was stressed to the limit, but the staff at the time was unbelievably proud of having risen to this disaster. In the meantime, the other nice cozy non-municipal hospitals each took just a few patients and, naturally, were not unduly stressed to provide care. When I arrived in June, there were still a few patients in the hospital from the previous Thanksgiving recovering from their burns. It is also worth remembering that there was no great pressure to send patients home from municipal hospitals during those times.

It may surprise doctors and patients today, but when I was a house officer and a young attending, city hospitals basically never forced a patient to be discharged. The net result was that in cold weather many patients who entered the hospital for quite legitimate illnesses would not just stay until they recovered completely, but would stay in the winter until the weather turned warmer.

In the Queens General Hospital medical units, which were basically one enormous ward with a triple row of beds, such patients were transferred out onto the porch. The porch was more like a solarium situated at the far end of the ward and separated from the ward by the utility/bath rooms and a couple of treatment rooms. In the early fall the porch might be tables and chairs with an occasional bed against the wall but by the end of winter, the porch would have wall to wall beds such that it was difficult to walk between any of the beds. Nonetheless, since it was heated, had sanitary facilities, and three meals a day, a significant number of people who had recovered but had no home to go to would stay on the unit until the weather turned more favorable. I might mention, since city hospitals in those days were chronically understaffed, that these recovered patients could also be very helpful to the nursing staff. They would feed patients, they would clean the floors, they might help make beds, and many of them, although they could not be forced to do so, generally made themselves useful on the unit. It is the commentary of the social services on the day that, for many of these people, the porch was a better place to be during the winter than out in the cold, cruel streets.

RESPIRATORS

The original machines to help patients breathe were iron lungs. I don't know how many people have ever seen a picture of an iron lung, but it is a tank big enough to hold the patient with a hole in one end with his head sticking out. Around his neck is a rubber foam cuff to make the tank airtight and a giant bellows, inflates and deflates the air in the tank, thereby squeezing the patient's chest and expanding the patient's chest, which is what causes air to enter and leave the patient's lungs. As a young intern, I had occasion to work in a hospital that treated Polio and that had dozens of patients in iron lungs. To this day, I remember the lovely young redheaded woman who came in with her daughter. Her child had a weak leg. The mother had a nasal voice. They both had new, acute Polio. In the course of the next six hours, the mother lost her voice completely, lost the ability to breathe, was placed in an iron lung, lost the ability to control any of her bodily functions and died of Polio. The child developed a completely paralyzed leg, but other than that, had no other symptoms and was discharged after several days to the distraught father, who took his daughter home to continue rehabilitation. It does not break my heart that the scourge of Polio is gone today.

ZINC

In 1945, a physician at the Wright Patterson Air Force Base, which I believe is in Ohio, published a short series of patients with slowly healing chronic wounds in which he felt the wounds healed more quickly when the patients were given extra zinc in their diet.

My father noticed this article and, seeing zinc as a basically harmless material, tried it on a few patients who had chronic ulcerated legs and found that they did indeed seem to improve. As time passed, he had a pharmaceutical company manufacture zinc sulfate in tablet form for him and began to give them for short periods to patients who didn't seem to be recovering well from their illness, as if their healing was somehow impaired. He got the general feeling that things did improve when these patients took a week or two of zinc, and while I was in medical school he and I discussed this. My medical school professors pooh-poohed the idea but, believing one's father, I also adopted the use of zinc in my practice and, through the years, had many patients who did seem to get better faster from various illnesses when they were given zinc. In more recent years I notice that the health food stores now carry zinc lozenges and zinc tablets and many people find them helpful.

I am not aware of any recent medical research on zinc in wound healing, but I do recall an article from Africa in which zinc seemed to both improve and prevent episodes in small malnourished children with chronic diarrhea. One of the problems in evaluating medical literature is the magic of the computer. To the best of my knowledge, no computerized analysis has been devoted to medical literature before approximately 1967. As a result, since finding literature older than that involves digging in the musty stacks of a library, there is very little recovered from the old days, even though much of those papers may well have contained useful medical information.

SPECIALTY BOARDS

Back in the mid 1930's, my father received a letter in the mail from an organization calling itself, rather grandly, the American Board of Internal Medicine. It proported to be a new specialty Board in the new specialty of internal medicine. At the time this happened the only existing specialty Board was a Board involved in ophthalmology, which seemed to most physicians as a very reasonable kind of specialty. This new specialty Board proposed, since my father had been trained at the Mount Sinai Hospital for two years after graduation, that he could be a charter member of this new wonderful organization, and all he had to do was fill out this application form and send them a check for $50. He scoffed at the idea and could not imagine why anyone would want to be a member of such an organization.

When I finished my residency training and began trying to obtain Board certification, the American Board of Internal Medicine was a two-part exam, each of them costing close to $1,000 and I found the examinations extremely difficult. My father thought it was hilarious that an organization that had offered him a charter membership, a founding membership in effect, for all of $50 was now grandly giving written and oral examinations to young physicians at impressive fees to offer them basically the same qualification.

At this time there is a whole spectrum of different specialty and even subspecialty Board certification examinations all at imposing fees, usually of at least $1,000 to certify young physicians in various disciplines. Through the years I have managed to garner specialty Boards in Internal Medicine, Emergency Medicine, and Geriatric Medicine. I have found all these examinations difficult and expensive.

NURSES

I

Nurses and doctors have worked as a team ever since Florence Nightingale. I say, without hesitation, that nurses have saved my ass many times, but I think of one in particular that will never leave me. I was a junior intern. During medical school summers, I found a way to work in hospitals to gain more experience and I worked as sort of an intern with the title of "clinical clerk". On this occasion, one of the jobs we had was to give babies an injection of an ounce or so of slightly salty water under their skins to combat dehydration. It was believed too difficult to keep an intravenous going in a baby, so this was the common method used to replace fluid when babies had vomiting or diarrhea or very high fever. One of my jobs was to do this procedure in babies in the nursery who required it, and I was called during the night to do this. The nurses in the nursery, in those days, were "baby nurses". They were not registered, trained nurses, but were mainly women who had learned how to take care of babies. As a result, the baby nurse on duty was not at all ready for me. I expected the syringe to be waiting with the salt water in it so that I could just turn the baby over, give it the injection and go back to sleep. I was quite irritable with her and kept saying, "Come on, get going, get the syringe filled, get me the alcohol." The alcohol, of course, was used to swab the skin before the injection was given. I might mention, in hospitals, in those days, the nurses kept the alcohol in bottles, but it was pigmented, usually with gentian violet, so it looked like nothing else. However, this was usually done by the nurse on each unit. After a delay, the nurse supervisor, who was a very highly trained nurse, appeared on the scene and just as she did, the baby nurse came back with the syringe of salty water and the cotton soaked in alcohol. I proceeded to get ready to give the baby the injection, when the nurse supervisor said, "Taste it." I said, "What do you mean?" She said, "Doctor, you didn't see the bottle that came out of. Before you give an injection, you want to know what you're injecting. Squirt a little on your hand and taste it. It should be slightly salty water." I squirted a little on my hand and tasted it. It was alcohol. Somehow, on this unit, the nurses had not colored all the alcohol and with all my talking about alcohol, the baby nurse had filled the syringe with uncolored alcohol and given it to me. If I had injected the baby with this, the baby would certainly have died. The supervising nurse's common sense vigilance had saved the baby's life and my ass. I have never forgotten that person. Today, of course, every one is trained to look three times at the medication they are injecting: once when they take it off the shelf, once when they load the syringe and once more just before they inject. It is a lesson well learned and can be, as in this case, a genuine lifesaver.

II

My Aunt Katie was a nurse trained at Mount Sinai Hospital in the 1910's. At Mount Sinai Hospital in the 1910's, a nurse was in charge of an entire ward, something like sixty patients. This meant not only giving the patients nursing care and medication and dressings and so forth and baths, but also it meant cleaning the floor and keeping the coal stove running on the unit. It also involved shaking down the ashes on the coal stove and shoveling them into a bucket and carrying the bucket to the dumper outside. This was done on a six and a half day workweek—six 12 hour shifts and one 6 hour shift, primarily so the nurses could go to church. I am not saying that everybody else in society didn't work much longer hours in those days, too, but when one thinks that this was routine nursing around WWI times and was taken for granted that the nurse could handle all of the nursing duties, plus all of the housekeeping duties on a ward, was routine, ordinary, represents a paradigm shift. In her later years in this changing world, my

Aunt Katie became a public health nurse in one of the rottenest neighborhoods in Flushing, where she made unaccompanied home visits, in her blue public health nurse uniform and her bag, to new mothers, newborn babies, sick people stuck at home and things of that nature. She was always totally safe in that regard. In recent years, I have learned that public health nurses must be accompanied by a guard, since they have been assaulted, robbed, and raped during home visits. I don't see myself as competent to comment upon the change in our society, but it has certainly changed public health nursing.

AMBULANCE ACTION

While I was working at that hospital, we made an ambulance call and came upon a baby who was gasping for breath. Resuscitating a baby requires special equipment that was not on the ambulance, so that all I could really do was hold an oxygen mask over the baby's face gently and pray a lot. I said to the ambulance driver, "GET US BACK TO THE HOSPITAL!" In this particular hospital, there was a toll bridge on the way to the hospital. Ordinarily, the ambulance would slow down, just a little, as it ran across the bridge, and it upset the toll collectors that this rather large vehicle would swish by them at what they saw as an unconscionable rate of speed. When they heard the siren and saw the ambulance coming, the toll bridge attendant decided to teach us a lesson and he put the toll bridge gate, a wooden barrier, down so we would have to stop at his booth. The driver, who realized I had a desperately ill baby, did not slow down at all. He went right through the wooden barrier and kept on going. The toll collectors sent the police after us, and the police caught up with us just as we were unloading this blue baby from the ambulance. They quietly got back in their vehicle and drove away.

ROOFING

When I was a clinical clerk, I often helped the anesthetist in the operating room who would let me do such things as start intravenous lines and assist in various phases of anesthesia. I should mention that the father of this anesthetist was the owner of a very large and successful roofing contracting company. Nonetheless, his son became a physician rather than go into the family business.

The story goes that the patient to be anesthetized was an enormously fat woman who hung over both sides of the operating table. Operating tables are quite narrow and I was concerned that if this woman moved she could fall and end up on the floor. Although she had a belt across her hips, it did not seem too substantial to me. The anesthetist began to try to put her to sleep with a mask supplying anesthesia gas over her nose and mouth along with an intravenous drug. She began to struggle, shaking her head back and forth, and rolling her body on the operating table. I became so concerned that she would fall that I literally threw my body across her to keep her from potentially falling. In this position, lying across her body, I heard the anesthetist mumbling over and over to himself. He was struggling to keep the mask on her nose and mouth while holding one arm with the intravenous still, and he was mumbling. I cocked my ear and what he was mumbling over and over was, "And I could have been in the roofing business. And I could have been in the roofing business."

PAIN

There are many, many stories in medicine about pain and suffering. I have already told you some, but here are several that I remember through the years. I made an ambulance call to a small cabin on stilts in the marshland in Jamaica Bay. To get to this cabin, you walked on precarious walkways, also on stilts, some of them rickety. As we walked toward this small house, the house was rocking. There would be a crash, and the house would shudder, and then there would be another crash and the house would shudder, and this continued as we approached. Upon entering, I found a large man (actually, I later learned, a football player) rolling in agony on the floor. He would roll one way until he banged into the wall and then he would roll back the other way until he banged into the wall. In this rickety cabin, this large man banging into the wall actually shook the whole building. A little history taking made it clear that he had a kidney stone, one of the more excruciating pains. I had a problem, since he was a very large man. If I relieved his pain completely with a potent narcotic, we would have to carry him on these rickety gangways, something that appeared to be impossible. On the other hand, he clearly was incapable of walking. I made a rapid calculation and gave him a half dose of morphine. Twenty minutes later, he was able, with difficulty, but able, to walk with us back to the ambulance and we took him off to the hospital.

For a period of time I had occasion to work in a hospice program. We treated patients who were terminal, at home. I came upon a charming elderly woman curled up in bed, in agony. Her daughter, with whom she lived, was utterly distraught that her mother never got out of bed, just lay in bed and moaned constantly. Upon history taking, I learned that she was being given an occasional dose of 25mg of demerol, a potent pain reliever, but a wholly inadequate dose. I arranged to get her oral dilaudid, a very potent pain reliever, in full doses. I got a phone call from the daughter the next day at suppertime. She said, "Doctor, I came home today. My mother was up and dressed and had cooked supper." The relief of this nice woman's pain had enabled her to become a functional person again, and for the next several months, until her cancer advanced and killed her. She was able to be helpful in the house and feel useful and not suffer so terribly. Cancer is often a chronic disease that can indeed be very painful and appropriate pain relief is something that should be offered to all patients. It has been pointed out by many authorities that cancer patients rarely become addicted and for terminal cancer patients, one would say that the addiction is irrelevant.

HOUSE CALLS

I

My father recalled a house call he made in Harlem, in the old days, in which he stopped on his way down the stairs from the apartment to tie his shoe. As he was tying his shoe, the apartment door burst open and the men in the family all came out. They had been watching for his appearance at the front door (watching out the window, of course) and when he did not appear in a reasonable length of time, they assumed he was being mugged on the stairway and rushed to his assistance.

II

While I'm on the subject of house calls, this is the one story in this book that is not mine or my father's. It is the story about curing a child's asthma by making a house call on his brother. It is a story that young physicians find particularly charming, and it was an experience of my good friend, Dr. Philip Shoob. Dr. Shoob was treating a small boy with intractable asthma. He went through the routine of eliminating allergens, getting rid of pets, getting rid of feather pillows, cleaning and dusting the room, taking all possible dusty objects out of the room, and yet the child continued to have episodes of asthma. At this point, he embarked upon skin testing, a very unpleasant procedure to a small child. He found that the child was allergic. In addition to house dust, which was expected, and some grasses and molds, he was allergic to citrus fruits. It was no big deal to eliminate citrus fruits from his diet and he did indeed improve a great deal, yet he continued to have episodes of asthma. One evening, the child's older brother had a fever and was acutely ill and the doctor made a house call. He was sitting on the sick child's bed examining him, when the mother was busy putting the younger child, the asthmatic child, to bed in the same room, since the boys shared a bedroom. He dimly heard, but it did not register, the mother saying to the child, "Here dear, take your pill and go to bed." Dr. Shoob finished his care of the older boy and was leaving when the dim recollection worked into the forefront of his mind and he said to the mother, "I didn't order any bedtime medication on the little fellow." The mother said, "Oh yes, I know, doctor. Every night, I give him a St. Joseph's baby aspirin to help him sleep." For those who are not in the know, the flavoring in St. Joseph's baby aspirin is orange. Eliminating this removed all the symptoms of the child's asthma.

III

Early in his practice, my father had occasion to make a house call in the Hotel Marquel, which to the best of my recollection became a building that was torn down secretively in the middle of the night. In any case, he went to the suite involved and was chatting with a gentleman about his complaints when a pretty young woman oozed into the room and walked unsteadily towards them. As she did, she said, "I must've had a wonderful time last night. I don't remember a thing." My father was unable to remember any of the man's complaints following this incident, and had to take his history all over again!

IV

My father recalled making house calls to shut-ins—people who really never got out at all. Not only would they request the house call, but they would give him a short shopping list so that he would have to come to the house not just with his medical bag, but with a bag of cheese, crackers and a bottle of milk when he arrived for the house call.

V

When I first started practice, I was willing to cover any doctor at any time for any thing. I made house calls half an hour from my office, if not more. I made house calls at any hour of the day or night. I would see anybody anywhere, since I was trying to build a practice. A Senior Internist, who I met, had allowed me to take some of his night calls. They were all very nice patients and I was happy to do it. One night, I was awakened with a call and I promptly dressed and left. As I walked into the house, the daughter, who was admitting me, mumbled under her breath, "Ahhh, the nighttime doctor." I began to realize that unless I wanted a life of my own, perhaps I should find another way of building my practice.

FEE SPLITTING

Another scourge in the old days in medicine was something called fee splitting. Fee splitting is certainly illegal today among doctors (I understand it is not illegal among lawyers), but what it represented is the family physician would diagnose, say appendicitis, and he would send the patient to the surgeon. The surgeon would do the operation and essentially half the fee would be handed back to the family physician for referring the case. In my father's early days, I have a feeling this was not illegal and, in fact, was utterly routine. As an intern, I can remember one physician talking to another about it at lunch and the first physician said, "In the Bronx, we split postage stamps." At one point, an extremely high-powered surgeon became a chief and yet he was felt to be a terrible surgeon. The net result was, my father told me, that he used to split 60% back to the referring doctor so he could get business. In any case, I resolved early on never to split fees and have always practiced that way. I would like to believe it no longer exists in medicine. Occasionally, in my early practice, until the word got out, I would get this sum of money, which I would credit to the patient's account quietly. Most patients never asked how they ended up with a credit on their accounts. The few that did, I told them that there had been a misunderstanding about the fee.

DOCTORS AS COLLEAGUES

The relationships between physicians have always fascinated me. For example, when I was a young doctor, many very nice senior internists would send me patients. Mostly, these were the patients who didn't pay their bills or who complained a lot or who, perhaps, were just cranky and irritable, but for whatever reason, the physician did not wish to care for them and would send them to me. The relations among physicians were very collegial and I would often have lunch with a group of physicians at one of the local hospitals. One particular physician, the one who I had covered previously on house calls, continued to send me patients and finally one day I said to him, "How can I pay you back?" His answer, "You can't." He said, "You're going to pay me forward." I said, "What do you mean?" He said, "When you get the chance to help a young colleague, you do so, just as I have tried to help you." It is a lesson I have never forgotten, and all my life, I have attempted to give young physicians a hand.

AMNESIA

A senior physician of my acquaintance developed a terrible bleeding ulcer. He was a lovely, European trained gentleman of the old school, and to watch him vomit his lifeblood was a terrifying and distressing experience. In those days, we were not yet rushing to do emergency surgery on these people, so I, and the gastroenterologist that I had called in consultation, were up until about 3:00 o'clock in the morning, washing his stomach out with ice water, and transfusing him. The entire time we did this, despite sedation, he gurgled and gasped and struggled and, when he could, screamed at us. I should mention the tube used for this purpose is essentially the thickness of a thumb, it is passed directly through the mouth to the stomach and it is a horrible experience. Finally, around 3:30 in the morning, we got the bleeding controlled, got him transfused back up, got him sedated quietly in bed, and we both left. I returned at 7:00 a.m. to see this man, who had just been shaved and had his hair combed, propped up in bed with a big smile. I asked him, "How do you feel?" He said, "Wonderful, this is great." I said, "How about last night?" He said, "What happened last night?" Amnesia is a wonderful thing. I didn't bother telling him how difficult the night had been for me. I might mention he recovered completely, and returned to practice for a quite a few more years.

DEATH

Physicians have, many times, a different view of life and death than the general population. Perhaps it is because of the suffering they see and the lingering, but I know many doctors who say they would rather not live with lingering and suffering. My father had occasion to treat an elderly physician who was suffering greatly and finally one evening he made a house call to find this physician dead, still holding the cyanide bottle in his hand. My father pronounced the patient, recorked the bottle and put it in his pocket, and issued a death certificate as "coronary thrombosis". I have a feeling that many suicides, in the old days, when suicide had such a hideous connotation, was mislabeled on many death certificates, as well as, many cancers. Even today, much of the statistics for death certificates that "authorities" are happy to quote, I believe, are filled with intrinsic errors. In any case, my father kept the bottle of cyanide. Years later, when he developed a brain tumor and terrible weakness, he threatened to use the bottle, and we, my brother, also a physician, and I, had a great deal of difficulty convincing him not to. He subsequently died of an acute coronary, as I have previously mentioned, and his secretary inherited the bottle. She didn't use it either and I do not know where it is now.

PLACEBO

A placebo is a fake. In medical research, it's a pill that looks like the real thing that you give to people without telling them in any way it's not the real thing and see if the real thing works any better than the fake thing. In practice, obviously, placebos are a different situation. A very common placebo is a sterile water injection. Sterile water is a little uncomfortable as an injection so that patients feel that they must be getting something and it is not uncommon if you feel a patient's pain is not real for whatever reason that you try a sterile hypo. Obviously, if the pain is relieved, it is not significant physical pain. There are other uses of placebos. My late father had phenobarbital, one-quarter grain tablets, in multiple different forms. The dose is so small that given once or twice a day, it is essentially innocuous for short-term use in an adult. It is amazing how many minor illnesses were cured with such pills. It is worthwhile to remember in this regard, that roughly 50% of patients will get well as long as the doctor's treatment does not make them worse. In other words, it's irrelevant what the treatment given is, since the illness is self-limited.

HUMILITY

No physician is right all the time. My father told me this story about right and wrong when I believed I was a very sharp intern.

For some twenty years, he cared for a nice woman who would come to the office whenever she was feeling ill. He would take a history, examine her, and write a prescription. She might return months later with a new complaint. He would ask how the prior illness responded, and the answer was always satisfactorily. This pattern of satisfactory medical care persisted for years. Then the patient appeared with a rapid pulse and shortness of breath. A physical examination detected the wet lungs and puffy ankles of heart failure. A prescription for digitalis was written. The patient returned ten days later feeling worse. When my father went to examine her, he found a string around her neck with an attached slip of paper. It was the digitalis prescription. "Why didn't you take this to the drug store and get the medicine?", he asked. "Doctor, every other time I put it around my neck and I got better. This time it didn't work." "Yes, indeed," my father said, "sometimes patients do get better because of what we do. Sometimes they get better in spite of what we do. Sometimes their recovery has nothing to do with us!" That is why research is carried out with placebos.

I, however, have a story about a placebo that I have never been able to reconcile. This is a nice woman that I took care of for some 40 years. Somewhere along the line, she had gotten the idea that she required B12 by injection to feel well and every month or so she would come to me demanding a B12 injection. Originally, I attempted the lecture that it didn't help and she insisted that she needed the injection and felt much better after she got it. Time passed, this pattern continued and I

was a little irritated with myself for what I saw as shady medical practice. Along came injectable polio vaccine—a red liquid in a vial. B12, I
might mention, is a red liquid in a vial. The next time she came in for
her B12 injection, I agreed, as I had been, took out the Polio vaccine,
filled the syringe of this red liquid right in front of her (she could not
read the label on the vial, of course), gave her the injection and sent her
merrily on her way. She called three days later. "Doctor," she said, "I
know that medicine seemed the same, but it didn't work." I recovered
quickly and said, "Maybe I didn't give you a big enough dose. Come
back and I'll give you another." This time I gave her the B12 red liquid
and I called her a few days later and she said, "Oh yes, that one worked
fine." I still have no explanation. I firmly believe I gave this woman no
clues that she was not getting a B12 injection and yet "it didn't work".

MORE ABOUT PAIN

I

One of the unique characteristics of pain is that only in a sympathetic way can we experience someone else's pain. Despite our best efforts we cannot feel their pain nor can we truly evaluate the depth of someone else's pain. We are all aware that some people seem to be stoical and either do not experience, or do not respond so much to pain. Others seem very sensitive and uniquely respond to pain. My father had an unusual relationship with pain. Perhaps a few stories will give the reader some insight into his feelings.

II

Drug addiction, and drugs in general, had started to become a scourge in our society by the time when my father required prostate surgery. The morning after surgery, I went in to see him and found him lying in bed in agony. He didn't have to say anything, obviously, the moment I looked at his face, I knew he was in agony and I said to him, "Let me get the nurse and get you a demerol injection." He said, "Don't you dare!" I said, "Why not? You're suffering." He said, "If I got one more of those wonderful injections I would <u>never</u> be able to stop." And he totally refused any additional pain relief. Interestingly, I have had demerol for operative pain and have found it to be nauseating, headachy, and only mildly relieving and I would never see it as something I would have the faintest interest in abusing. Apparently, my father's metabolism was very different from mine.

III

It is a beautiful summer day and we are standing on the elevated platform outdoors at 125th Street and Broadway. I look over at my father and on the side of his neck is a large black beetle. I grab the beetle to pull it off his neck. Its jaws are locked on the skin of his neck such that it pulls up the skin. The beetle finally lets go and I throw it off the platform. My father slowly turns and looks at me in a puzzled way. It was clear that he did not experience the beetle's pinch on his neck as something painful, nor apparently, had he actually felt the beetle at all on his neck until I attempted to pull it off.

IV

It is another beautiful summer day and I am quite young. We are standing in shallow water at Lake Mahopac in front of my grandfather's house. There are several large rocks in the shallow water, and my father wishes to move them to be resting partly on the shore and partly in the water as a support for more earth. He reaches under a large rock with both hands and goes to pick it up. Unbeknownst to him, there is a broken bottle under the rock. Before he appreciates the sharp edge, it cuts his finger. He takes his hand out of the water and holds the skin of the middle finger. The flesh on the front surface of the finger has been peeled away, so the bone and tendon are visible in the bottom of the wound. He says not a word, wraps his other hand around the injured finger and quietly walks down the road to Dr. Stacey's office. He returns within the hour with a large bandage. The finger heals uneventfully, but is somewhat deformed. I was too young at the time to discuss pain with him but clearly he was unaware at first that he was cutting his finger on this broken bottle, and made not a sound either before or after the injury.

V

As a teenager, I was quite strong. There was a porcelain-handled faucet in my aunt's bathtub. When I shut the faucet off, it continued to drip. Consequently, I leaned on the faucet, which broke, and the sharp edges of the break slashed into the palm of my hand quite deeply. Oddly enough he wound hardly bled. Upon examining the wound though, tendon and artery, and vein as well as muscle, were clearly visible in the depths of the wound. None of the structures appeared to have been injured. My father was nearby and he told me that this would have to be stitched. He decided we would go to the office nearby of Dr. Nina Lief, a very nice woman who was a friend of the family. While my father let me squeeze his hand, Dr. Lief put four or five stitches to pull the flap back together. Despite my best efforts to be brave, putting the needle through the skin to sew the skin edges together was extremely painful. Tying the knot to pull the skin edges together was excruciating. In fact, the wound itself hardly hurt, while after the repair, it was quite painful for the next day or two.

ANESTHESIA

While we're on the subject of pain, I can recall vividly a unique use of special anesthesia for a painful condition. My father called me into the office, I was eleven or twelve, to assist him. In those days he had no full time medical assistant and often practiced alone with his patients. The patient in question had an enormous carbuncle on the back of his neck. For those who do not know what a carbuncle is, it is a giant boil with multiple heads. The back of the neck is a particularly bad situation for the carbuncle because the anatomy is such that each individual head must be drained to get a cure. This was, of course, all in the days before antibiotics and a surgical drainage was the only cure. Today, of course, surgical drainage would be combined with antibiotics and the cure might be much faster. Because of the multiple heads of the carbuncle a very large incision is required to get adequate drainage of all areas. The carbuncle is already "as sore as a boil" and the added pain of opening this with a scalpel would truly be excruciating. My father sat the patient down in his ENT chair, a substantial iron tubular chair with a headrest and arm rests. In front of him, he put a tray supported by a Mayo stand, nothing more than a supporting arm on legs. On that Mayo stand he put a sterile towel. In front of that stand he put a second Mayo stand with another sterile towel. In those days medical instruments were sterilized by boiling them in an electric sterilizer, a large shiny nickel-plated contraption the size of a breadbox with a tray and several inches of boiling water. My father proceeded to raise the lid of this large shiny boiling sterilizer, reach in with a forceps and start removing instruments. He first took out his scalpel and put it on the towel. He then proceeded to remove several more instruments and put them on the towel. The patient during this, with this array of instruments in front of him, became more and more anxious looking and little sweaty and pale. At this point, my father handed me a large wad of sterile gauze and continued to remove instruments from the sterilizer. At one point, I realized that he had removed one-half of an obstetrical forceps blade, an enormous shiny, curved tortuous-looking instrument, but one that even I realized had no utilization in draining a boil. At approximately that moment, the patient's distress overcame him and he fainted dead away pitching forward onto the first mayo stand. My father grabbed the scalpel and immediately opened the boil. I put the wad of gauze on and as the patient came out of his faint, the procedure had already been accomplished. Not verbal anesthesia exactly, but certainly very fine anesthesia for the case involved.

FRACTURED HIPS

Despite our best treatment, fractured hips are a curse of old age. The sad statistic was that close to half of all elderly people who fractured their hips were dead within a year. There are a few stories about fractured hips from the old days however, that I think are worthy of illustration.

I am in intern in the Jewish Memorial Hospital in upper Manhattan. The ambulance brings an elderly gentleman to our emergency room with, literally, a shattered hip. The upper end of his thighbone is in multiple pieces, and he is in severe pain and looks a bit shocky. In those days nobody rushed to repair these injuries. It was seen as so difficult that the standard treatment was to put the patient in traction to realign fragments. Once in a more physiological natural position, surgery would be considered to put in the hardware and fix the fragments in position. This is distinctly different from today, when emergency surgery as soon as the patient can be stabilized and brought to the operating room is the more common procedure. We put this man to bed and I elected to put him up in the most elaborate traction called balanced traction. This involved a framework over the bed to support a very elaborate series of pulleys, ropes, splints and hinges to try to apply proper traction on the hip. It took me several hours to install this elaborate framework and attach it to the patient properly. When I was done, both the patient and I were quite exhausted and he was still in considerable pain. I gave him a very small amount of pain medication. I left to perform other duties. Hours later I came back to find the gentleman in his traction, head of the bed elevated, a light on, his hair combed, his glasses on, and he was busy reading the New York times.

When I inquired, he assured me that the pain was almost gone. I congratulated myself on a wonderful approach to this man's injury and expected the orthopedists to operate on him relatively soon. We x-rayed his hip each day, and the fragments continued to be quite out of position. The surgeon felt that surgery was not yet indicated. Each day he looked a little more tired. After two or three days, he began to get a little short of breath. This rapidly progressed such that on the fifth hospital day he died. An autopsy disclosed that the circulation in the lungs was filled with globules of fat. This fat had become dislodged from the bone marrow in his fractured hip. It had spread into his veins and the veins had carried it to his lungs. He died from what was called massive fat embolus. This is one of the complications even now of major fractures of bone.

Ada

Some fractured hips do not require immediate surgery and are not that painful. The case in point is that involving my elderly Aunt Ada. She sustained a fall and noticed a pain in her hip. X-ray revealed a crack completely across the upper end of the hip. This crack however, was exactly that. The bones were not displaced in anyway. Her surgeon said to her that he wished to operate, and put a couple of large screws across the crack area so the bones could not come apart until they healed. The thought of surgery was very unpleasant to my aunt and consequently she asked the surgeon what were her other choices, since she did not wish an operation. He replied that she could go to bed for about six weeks and put no weight on the hip and perhaps it would heal. However, he warned her of the very real risks in someone in her age group (she was over 80 at the time) staying in bed continuously for this length of time. She decided that that's what she wished to do. She promptly obtained some assistance in her apartment, and went home to bed. She returned to the surgeon six weeks later. An x-ray revealed that the bone had indeed healed without incident. I might mention this is never a recommended procedure, but in her case it did indeed workout very well. She never had any further trouble with the hip, and lived many years thereafter.

MORE AMBULANCE CALLS

I have mentioned a few ambulance calls, but there are always more that come to mind. While I was an intern, we rode the ambulance in those days (physicians, of course, no longer do). I was called to the roof of an apartment house. The elevator was not running and the police led me to the elevator shaft access door and there, on the roof of the building was a seven or eight year old boy, lying on top of the elevator with his thigh amputated, approximately in the middle, and the leg lying along side him. His leg had somehow become caught in the main steel cable that raised and lowered the elevator and went up over the pulley under the roof at which point the leg was amputated and considerably crushed. There was a great deal of grease on the stump, but no bleeding of any significance. Between the crushing and the normal retraction of injured vessels, the bleeding was controlled. The boy was, of course, pale, sweaty and shocky. We were some three blocks from the hospital and I decided to put a sterile towel over the thigh stump, bring the leg and go immediately to the hospital. The surgeon elected not to attempt a reattachment because of the grossly contaminated nature of the wound and the enormous crushing of the leg muscles. He healed satisfactorily for an artificial limb, however, and made an uneventful, but sad, recovery.

FAMILY

I

There is an old medical adage to the effect that a physician, who cares for himself, has a fool for a doctor and a bigger fool for a patient. Frequently, physicians believe that this unwillingness to treat, should also extend to families. On the other hand, there is a terrible temptation, since physicians all have very large egos, to feel that you can do a better job since, of course, you know your family better than anyone else. I recall vividly a colleague, now deceased, who treated his daughter's bellyache casually to the point where she ended up with a ruptured appendix and a very prolonged convalescence. I have a feeling a patient in the same circumstances would have gone to surgery much sooner. In fact, although I did not delay, my own son, as a teenager, had a bellyache and the surgeon decided to procrastinate during the day. Interestingly, his bellyache, despite an elevated white count and classical clinical signs, went away by evening and he was not operated on and still has his appendix.

II

As a young physician, I felt comfortable taking care of my children's minor illnesses and was available to them at any time. I also used to keep powdered oral antibiotics for children in the house at all times so a child that was acutely ill could get immediate treatment rather than having to run to a drug store. My four-year-old son woke me one night to tell me that he had a terrible pain in his ear. I got up, got my ear examining machine, called an otoscope, examined both ears and sure enough the ear he complained of was indeed acutely inflamed. I mixed up a vial of the powdered penicillin to make a tasty strawberry flavored medicine, gave him two teaspoonfuls, gave him a baby aspirin (in those days we were still giving aspirin to children, such of course is not true anymore) cuddled him for a few minutes and carried him back to bed, tucked him in and sat with him for a couple of minutes to calm him down, assured him that he would feel better and went back to bed. He awoke me thirty minutes later shaking me and saying, "It didn't work, Dad."

III

Many years ago when my children were very small, I served for several years as the county medical examiner. One of my more difficult jobs involved home visits. Periodically, I would get a call at 8:00 or so in the morning to visit a home where a baby had been found dead in its crib. I would enter a house in which the parents were stunned and almost mute and tormented grandparents and other family members would be sitting around not knowing what to do or what to say. The baby, often a totally darling obviously well cared for child, would be found in the crib solidly dead, probably having died at 2:00 or 3:00 in the morning. These sudden infant deaths were not at all explained in those days, nor is there a total agreement even today on what the cause might be. After evaluating the situation, I would inform the family that an autopsy would be done and the body would be removed to the morgue. This did not add to anyone's comfort, my own included, but it was the routine at the time. Sadly, despite the best efforts of the medical examiner's office, it was unusual to find anything remarkable during the autopsy. Once in a while, an unrecognized congenital heart situation would make it easier to inform the family that we had found a cause of death, but more often the autopsy revealed nothing of note. We would really have no documentable cause of death. Each time I did this, particularly when the babies and families appeared to be lovely middle-class people and the child was obviously adored, I carried a significant burden out of the house. Often on those nights, I would find myself lying awake in my quiet home listening to my small children breathe.

IV

I was beeped one afternoon with my home number. When I called back, my wife, in a very stressed tone, said, "Please come home right now!" I said, "What's the matter?" She said, "Please come home right now." I left the office and went home to find her attached to the sewing machine. She been sewing using the electric sewing machine and somehow had driven the needle through her finger. The needle went through the nail, through the bone of the tip of the finger and protruded on the other side and she was sitting in her chair at her machine, looking very upset, as could be imagined. She had, fortunately, been able to reach the telephone to beep me and to answer the phone when I called back, but she was truly pinned. However, I realized immediately that the needle can be removed from the machine, so I was able to release the needle so she could at least get away from the machine, but she still, of course, had the needle through her finger. After considerable thought about the pain situation, I said to her that I think getting it out quickly will be the best method. She agreed with some hesitation (it's amazing what wives will put up with) and I proceeded to sterilize the needle and the surrounding skin with alcohol, hold her finger firmly, take an ordinary pair of pliers and in a trice, remove the needle. The wound healed uneventfully, and in fact, I never even got an x-ray. The only treatment rendered other than a bandage was to give her a tetanus booster, although the chances of tetanus on a home sewing needle do seem very slim.

V

As a small child, my youngest brother had a cystic development in the tear duct of his eye. As a result, the tear duct was blocked and the eye was constantly watery and puffy. My parents naturally took him to an ophthalmologist, who proceeded to attempt to probe the tear duct. On a toddler, this was an extremely tiny structure and what happened was my parents and my brother became very upset. Finally, my father said to my mother, "I'll take care of it." He proceeded to massage the effected corner of my brother's eye everyday and sure enough after several weeks the blockage opened and the tearing stopped. To the best of my knowledge the eye continues to be fine to this day.

VI

One day, my teenage daughter, Susan, developed nausea and vomiting and was very miserable. I promptly gave her some anti-nauseant. In a relatively short time, she continued to vomit and complain bitterly, so I gave her some more anti-nauseant. She continued to vomit and complain further, so I gave her some more anti-nauseant and shortly thereafter she turned green while sitting at the kitchen counter and passed out. Luckily, her siblings were able to catch her. She was uninjured, but clearly heavily overdosed with a potent anti-nauseant.

The sad fact is that when one loves the patient, one's judgment may indeed be impaired and foolish decisions result.

DRUGS

In this regard, perhaps I should give some thought to the interesting concerns about drugs, but before attacking drugs, one must first think of the placebo effect. A placebo is a harmless medication that can have only an affect upon the patient's belief system and all research studies of drugs are, of course, not only accompanied by placebos, but by placebos that appear to be exactly the same as the active drug and both the patient and the investigator have to be blinded to the realities. A very powerful placebo, in years past, was a sterile hypodermic, an injection of sterile water and many patients expressed great improvement in multiple conditions, particularly, painful conditions, upon receiving a sterile hypo. We now know, of course, that merely injecting into the skin can result in the body producing morphine-like substances that do, indeed, diminish pain. Some believe that is part, at least, of the reason for the success of acupuncture.

NARCOTIC PARANOIA

The bureaucrats in the Department of Health foolishly believed that physicians are the major source of abused narcotics. Consequently, they have saddled physicians with special triplicate forms for narcotic prescriptions. Supposedly the state gets a copy of every prescription so they could ride herd on abusive doctors. As a result of this, anxious physicians worried about being branded an abuser and often cut back on narcotic prescriptions. In my practice, I wrote perhaps one or two triplicate forms a month.

After several years of using these prescription forms, I took a part-time job with Visiting Nurse Service of New York, as a physician in their hospice program. The hospice program treated patients who were not expected to live longer than six months. They were maintained in their home with multiple visits by nurses and various therapists. My job basically was to make decisions about pain control, and write the triplicate prescriptions. Since these were all patients with very limited prospects, I had no hesitation in prescribing impressive amounts of potent medication. I found myself writing more than a dozen prescriptions for significant amounts of narcotics for many patients each week. This continued for several months. I was forced to put in an emergency order with the Department of Health for more prescription blanks, which were promptly supplied. I left the job a few months later and went back to my one or two prescriptions a month. I never heard a word from the Department of Health. Clearly paranoia over triplicate prescriptions is unwarranted.

PHYSICIANS

This is going to be a group of stories about physicians—training, practicing, hospital relationships, personal relationships, and collegial relationships...

I

It is, I believe, an open secret that physicians tend to be the most individualistic, egocentric population group in America. There are those that believe that the modern generation of doctors is somewhat more team oriented and less looking for the star quality in themselves, however, I must say that I have not found that to be so. Young doctors are, however, much more capable and happy working together in small groups, two or three collegial groups, while physicians in my fathers day and in mine, tended to be more and more solo.

II

Along with this individualist frame of mind is the joy of second-guessing other physicians, it is so routine at social gatherings to find physicians critiquing diagnoses and treatment of others. This is true despite the fact that all the malpractice insurers warn physicians to be discreet in their criticisms of their colleagues. By the same token, young physicians particularly enjoy making streetcar diagnoses, that is looking at people across the aisle and making such comments as "look at those eyes, obviously hyperthyroid" or "look at swelling of the legs, obviously renal or cardiac". Although much of this can be seen as sharpening one's diagnostic skills, most of it is also a form of one-upping, or second-guessing other physicians.

III

While we're on the subject of physician's egos, every doctor likes to make a good decision and obviously likes to take credit for it. I recall the case of the eighty-year-old patient in the nursing home who was convalescing from a fractured hip. During the convalescence, which took several weeks, his wife, an equally elderly woman, would visit him and the two of them would get into terrible verbal battles. At a certain point, it came to the attention of the social service department that it did not appear that he would be able to go home with her. We all agreed that he could not go home to live alone. It became more and more clear, as the battles escalated, that his wife would not accept him.

Since his discharge was imminent, I was asked to evaluate the patient. He assured me that he had a solution but did not care to share it. He seemed so confident that I approved his discharge, without knowing exactly what his plan was. The discharge planners were totally skeptical, but I trusted the patient. In effect, my reputation became a hostage to his discharge. He solved the problem by going home to live with his ninety-five year old mother who welcomed him home very happily, and was able to keep house for him.

IV

When my father was a young house officer at the Mount Sinai Hospital, he was somewhat isolated from the senior staff of the institution and was, of course, economically vastly inadequate. Nonetheless one day, he received an invitation to dinner from one of the senior medical attendings. It turned out that the dinner was at the luxurious 5th Avenue apartment of the brother of the physician in question. Present at a relatively small dinner party along with the physician and his wife, the brother and his wife and an elderly aunt or two, was a most winsome young woman, the niece of the physician, that is the daughter of his brother. She was quite lovely and very well spoken, but at a dinner table there was, of course, not much opportunity for any real interaction. At the end of the evening, the men separated from the women and went into the library of the apartment for brandy and cigars. I might mention, apartment is quite an inadequate word for these residences that were frequently more than one story within large 5th Avenue masonry towers. As the evening progressed, my father was asked for his opinion of the young lady and he said rather carefully that she seemed very nice indeed and was very pretty. At which point, her father said, "You know, my brother and I would very much like to see her married and she comes with a dowry of $50,000." I must mention that in the early 1920's, $50,000 was indeed a great deal of money. It is worth remembering that the average hard working man was lucky to earn $5.00 a day. Obviously in this context, such a sum was extremely generous and it made my father curious. At some point he was able to stammer out puzzlement on the specifics of such an arrangement and the reason therefore—there was a very long and profound silence and finally the girls uncle stated carefully that she was a lovely, lovely girl, but she was just a little bit pregnant.

V

My father and mother went to his twenty-fifth medical school reunion, and my mother, at least, had a perfectly lovely time. My father had worked so hard to support himself during medical school that he had little time for social life, but everybody was extremely nice to my mother and multiple members of the class regaled her with stories with how my father always had all the answers. In fact, he had actually taught his own classmates bacteriology since he had a master's degree in bacteriology before he attended medical school and as such he was apparently better qualified to teach it then anyone at that time on the Harvard Medical School staff. When it came time for his 50th reunion, my mother had passed on, but I offered to go with him. He said he was not planning to go to the reunion and saw no reason to make the trip. "None of my classmates will be there," he said.

VI

I have attended my 25th, my 40th and my 45th reunions, as well as some earlier ones, and found them all most enjoyable. It is amazing how sharing those four difficult years in medical school is a bonding experience that literally lasts a lifetime and I would pick up as if we had met yesterday with classmates that I had literally not seen or spoken to in 25 or 30 years. For those who have misgivings about attending any advanced reunion, I would strongly urge them to reconsider, whatever their social position in the class at the time of graduation at an advanced reunion, 25 years or more, such differences are irrelevant, and my experience has been that everybody has a perfectly wonderful time.

HOSPITAL PRIVILEGES

It will be a complete surprise to young doctors today, but when both my father and I were at our busiest practice years, hospital privileges were close to impossible in the New York area. Teaching hospitals reserved their spaces for those who would either give money or a great deal of free time or send an enormous number of patients. In addition, for many years when I first started practicing, hospitals were so jammed that they were not even interested in very many patients and that was not a selling point in terms of getting staff privileges. For many years, I was able to obtain staff privileges at the Jamaica Hospital only by giving three months of full service time in which I made rounds six and seven days a week with the house staff, without any salary. This was a wonderful learning experience for me. The chairman of my service, Dr. Ernest Keet, Jr., was a wonderfully competent and educational kind of leader who offered to give the five or six of us a great deal of attention and support. When Dr. Keet retired to practice in Saranac Lake, New York, my feelings and respect for him were so strong that I considered following him there to practice and, in fact, corresponded on the matter for a period of time.

My elderly aunt, who lived in Port Washington, became a patient and inquired of me if I could, if the need arose, hospitalize her in North Shore Hospital. I informed her that this was impossible since I did not have staff privileges. In point of fact, I had applied repeatedly to both Long Island Jewish and North Shore Hospitals when they first opened in the 1950's, and had not been accepted at either staff. My aunt was incensed, picked up the phone, and called a Port Washington High School classmate who I later learned was, quite literally, the President of the Board of North Shore Hospital. In a one-minute conversation, she informed him that her nephew needed staff privileges at North Shore Hospital and they were awarded to me within two months. I guess it's what we all learn—unfortunately it's often not what you know, but who you know that determines your success in life.

CRIMINALLY NEGLIGENT HOMICIDE

As I am in the process of writing this book, I received a terrible jolt while watching the television news this morning. A pompous prosecuting attorney in California was bragging that he had indicted seven professionals, doctors and dentists, on the criminal charge of manslaughter in the care of patients. His self-righteousness that this was protecting society made me nauseated. The thought that a professional, honestly trying to help a sick person has hanging over his head the specter that if a patient dies, the doctor would be seen not nearly as negligent, but as criminally so, seems overwhelmingly stupid to me. Medicine in all its scientific rigor, continues to be an art as well as a science and not only do we not have all the answers, we don't even remotely have all the questions. The thought that the physician can prevent all deaths is not only foolish, but narrow to an extreme. Several years ago, a physician in New York misidentified a feeding tube and was convicted of criminally negligent homicide and at the time I found that ridiculous. Although we would all like to always do our best for every patient, that does not indicate that 1) we will never ever be honestly mistaken, or 2) that despite the most careful scrupulous attention to all details, people will still die. I think I remember a line from an old M*A*S*H episode in which Hawkeye expresses his distress that despite his best efforts young men were dying. Despite anyone's best efforts, all of us will eventually die. The thought somehow that a physician doing honest care can be seen as having criminal negligence is just unbelievable to me and one wonders what this trend might lead to.

OBSTETRICS

I

Obstetrical stories are in many ways the most fun in medicine. Obviously delivering a baby is a joy to patient and doctor alike and the occasional tragedies, although extremely troubling, hardly stack up against the usual wonderful results. I recall a beastly hot night when I was a medical student spending the summer at the old Rockaway Beach Hospital, a non-air conditioned building. I had scrubbed in on a forceps delivery with one of the senior obstetricians who specialized in delivering using a modality called saddle block anesthesia. This is a particular kind of low spinal anesthesia in which the pregnant woman really does have complete relief of any significant pain. Consequently, there is not a great deal of pressure on the patient to push the baby out and frequently outlet forceps are necessary. A big advantage of the procedure is that any obstetrical tears that may need repair can be done painlessly and the patient can still walk because the very low spinal anesthesia is so carefully localized to the obstetrical delivery area. We had just finished delivering a healthy baby of a woman and had put her back to bed. The doctor and I and the nurses were sitting in the nurses' station finishing up paperwork on the case and chatting idly when from the patient's room came earth-shattering screams of pain and horror. We all immediately ran to the room. As we entered the room, the woman was standing just back from the open window wearing literally a johnny opened up the back and a peroneal pad held by a small belt. The moment we entered, she stopped screaming and climbed back into bed. The obstetrician said, "What were you doing?" "Oh," she said, "just getting my new mink coat."

II

I recall vividly the troubled woman who came to my father newly pregnant, upset about the extra nipples on her chest. In the normal human, a nipple may appear anywhere from the armpit to the groin, along a pair of lines called the "nipple lines". The vast majority of people have two nipples in the usual location. This woman had two nipples in the usual location, two nipples quite a bit higher, almost to the armpit and two nipples down almost on the level with her bellybutton. As this pregnancy progressed, it became apparent that all six nipples also had attached breast tissue and toward the end of her pregnancy, she was indeed a formidable young woman. More distressing is that after delivery, she found she could nurse at all six nipples. Although her baby was well nourished, the mess that the oozing, lactating nipples made on her clothing was something very upsetting to her. What my father told her, I remember, at one visit is she really should have had multiple births since she had all these nipples, but she did not think that was very funny.

OVERCOAT DOCTORS

My father, having been trained at Harvard Medical School and Mount Sinai Hospital in medicine, one would suspect that he was somewhat more medically sophisticated than many of the other physicians of the day. It is worth remembering that in the early 1900's, America was peopled with some pretty atrocious medical schools, which were mostly closed by an investigative intervention ending in the Flexner Report. In any case, he had a great disdain for what he called "overcoat" doctors. I recall this conversation when I was a medical student since he had in one of the bottom drawers in one of his cabinets a stethoscope with a big flat diaphragm some three inches across. It did not appear to be an obstetrical stethoscope and I asked him what it was for. He said, "Oh, those are for the overcoat doctors." I said, "What do you mean?" He said, "With that stethoscope, you can examine the patient's heart through their overcoat and still hear it." I tried it and indeed he was right. It was not very clear sounds, but you could indeed with a large diaphragm stethoscope hear the heart through multiple layers of clothing. Physicians, for those of you who are not aware, are always trained to put a stethoscope on bare skin today. In olden times, and there are some darling cartoons of this method, physicians would put their ear to the patient's bare skin, since the stethoscope had not been invented, or sometimes would put a very clean towel on the patient and then their ear to the towel. Today, if your physician does not put his/her stethoscope on bare skin you are being given a second rate examination and should govern yourself accordingly.

THE NATURAL HISTORY
OF DISEASE

Both my father and I were classically trained in the days when patients stayed in the hospital until they were well. This gave the doctor in training a particularly unique perspective on how patients reacted to an illness. A patient with pneumonia, in the days before antibiotics, would be sick for many weeks, have a crisis, and if they survived would usually recover. There were of course, multiple chances for complications or even death along the way. After antibiotics, the crisis was usually avoided and the patient would ordinarily begin to recover fairly rapidly, at first, but then frequently slow down in their recovery as the lung damage cause by the pneumonia took time to heal. The vast majority of common illnesses like heart failure, abdominal problems, skin infections, and respiratory infections, all have a kind of usual and ordinary progress as they respond to treatment. Patients staying in the hospital for all the recovery time, gave the young physicians the opportunity to see what the normal, usual, ordinary kind of convalescence should be and was a valuable learning experience. Today, unfortunately, patients are sent home from the hospital "quicker and sicker" and young physicians in training don't get to see how further progress develops. Medical schoolteachers make many attempts to have patients return to give young doctors an observation opportunity, but in truth the system in most places does not work too well. Consequently, young physicians have a very poor understanding of the natural recovery from many illnesses and as a result have trouble deciding whether a patient complaining on the telephone is doing as one would expect, better than one would expect or worse than one would expect. From this point of view, although very expensive, longer hospitalization has very real value in a teaching program. The modern day exaggeration of the importance of cost over health has many negatives in terms of the best care and the best medical education. Perhaps elsewhere in this book, I may get a chance to expound on this more fully.

MISTAKES HAVE BEEN MADE

For some 40 years, I have served as an expert witness in medical malpractice cases mostly, although not entirely, on behalf of the defense. My view of these cases has always been that a full understanding by both sides of the issue should result in a sensible and rapid solution, either abandonment of the case or settlement. This activity has never been a large part of my practice but through the years the cases do add up. Perhaps, however, the phrase "expert witness" is misleading because in the 40 years I have actually had to appear in court on such cases, on behalf of one side or the other, 20 times. This indicates that the vast majority of such cases are either abandoned or settled prior to or sometimes during trial.

The cases I have reviewed generally come under rather simple scenarios….a failure to diagnose a serious disease quickly or a failure to properly treat. Failure to diagnose, particularly in cases of cancer, is very upsetting to juries and such cases are mostly settled. For example, a patient will develop breast cancer and then recall that she saw some other doctor a year earlier so he must have missed the cancer. This is a simplistic and frequently inaccurate conclusion, but the thought of delay in a cancer diagnosis is so powerful to a jury that most defense experts advise against going to trial. The truth is that most cancers are the ultimate chronic disease and it is very difficult to show that delay has resulted in a significant change in the outcome.

In fact, very recently there has been a lot of medical controversy about the actual value of mammograms in making early diagnoses of breast cancer, but obviously lay people on juries will assume that any delay, sometimes even a week or two, somehow affects the outcome of the situation.

In general, I am far more disturbed when I review cases that involve criticism of a course of treatment and a poor outcome. The idea that a judgment made in good faith that does not produce a cure must in some way be negligent is totally alien to me. I have great difficulty seeing an error in a situation of that sort when the judgment seems appropriate at the time under the circumstances.

My father practiced medicine for 53 years and never carried malpractice insurance of any kind. In his early days the concept did not exist in society and nobody expected perfection on the doctor's part. Toward the end of his practice life the specter of malpractice had been raised in society, but by that time he had abandoned any hospital practice, was only involved in a private office practice mostly with his long term patients, and saw no need to spend money for malpractice insurance. I, on the other hand, have always carried this insurance and its cost through the years has gone up astronomically. My first original premium was less then $100 per year.

One of the reasons for my father's freedom from this scurge was that patients at one time seemed aware that medicine was a combination of an art and an inexact science and perfection was just not to be expected. In more recent times it is clear that society sees medicine as an exact science, capable of preventing death, and always batting 1000. This concept is ridiculous but, nonetheless, is one that the trial lawyers foster and are making a very good living on.

The concept of never being wrong also results in physicians attempting to protect themselves from any charges of negligence. Consequently, they order repeated batteries of laboratory and x-ray studies and frequently obtain multiple consultations. This behavior particularly is noted in hospital practice and I am convinced that this self-protective behavior on the part of physicians adds an enormous amount to the costs of medical care. The underlying cause of all this behavior is the attempt by trial lawyers to divert large sums of money to their bank accounts. In a way, the trial lawyers activities represent an enormous tax, not just on physicians for malpractice premiums, but on society paying the, what I believe to be excessive, costs of over protective medical care.

In recent years government has also gotten involved in the search for total error-free medicine. One activity the State engages in involves statistical follow-up of the outcomes, for example, of cardiovascular surgery specific to each hospital and even each cardiovascular surgeon. Since the statistics involved become public records discernable to anyone who wishes to look for it, cardiovascular surgeons are forced to practice protective behavior. In New York State, this basically translates into every surgeon looking only for the easiest safest cases to operate on. In New York State, particularly, really desperately ill patients requiring cardiac surgery may have to go out of state to find a surgeon willing to approach their problem because of the fear of a bad result branding the surgeon as somehow incompetent. What we are seeing here is one of the results of unintended consequences. The State wishes to improve the caliber of cardiac surgery, but in the process they are sentencing the most desperately ill patients to having difficulty finding anyone willing to operate on them. This is an extremely troubling situation to me since I have, in my practice days, had to send patients to Dr. DeBakey in Houston for them to obtain surgery. The cost of an air ambulance trip to Houston, in effect, is added to the patient's cost for surgery, in his travels to find a surgeon willing to operate. Looking back, this is a rather long chapter and I realize that I have developed a tiresome tirade. I do not see malpractice lawsuits as the way to improve the quality of our medical care or the outcomes of our treatment. In fact, I see the legal antagonistic system as a very poor way to resolve disagreements concerning medical or surgical treatment.

EUTHANASIA

Earlier in this book I promised that I would get to talk about euthanasia. It is commonly accepted in our society that people will mercifully kill their beloved pets when their existence reaches the point of pain, misery, and suffering, rather than loving companionship. There are certainly people who love their pets more than most of their fellow humans and yet large numbers of people, obviously, openly accept euthanasia for failing animals.

Euthanasia for human beings is, of course, a more difficult subject. Physicians who have seen far more people dwindle and die than the average population, I have found, can often readily accept the thought of, if not active euthanasia, at least a lack of enormous attempts to maintain life at all costs. Our technology today can literally keep a dead-brained person alive for years with breathing machines and parenteral feedings. The newspapers will periodically print an obituary of someone who has been in a coma in a nursing home for 20 and 30 years before they finally slip away.

I personally feel that this assiduous attention to a living existence rather than a peaceful death is overdone. I accept, of course, that many people's personal standards or religious beliefs force them to totally reject this viewpoint and I have no reason to feel that this is not their honestly held belief. I do not hold this belief and, in fact, have taken all the legal steps to make certain that my basically terminally ill body will not be kept alive unnecessarily to promote lingering, suffering, and pointless expense. In this regard, the word expense raises hackles with many since putting a price on the value of life is such a difficult philosophical, ethical, moral, and religious decision with lots of legal overtones. On the other hand, in terrible accidents it is possible for the insurance industry and the courts to put a price on the value of life and this does not seem to have such terrible ethical, moral consequences in society. In many ways, I see society's attitude toward this as a total denial, acting as if there is no such thing as death.

DYING

There are many vignettes about dying. There are many times when the death of a patient has a profound effect upon young physicians in training. I will allude to a few of them in this chapter, but I think I would like to first talk about physicians assisting patients in ending their lives.

I

I have always told patients, and other doctors, that I didn't go to medical school to kill people. On the other hand, I am not completely convinced that everybody who is dying needs or wants every last potential intervention that could be dreamed up applied to their terminal care. I can think of many times when the kindest, most therapeutic intervention for a dying patient would be an appropriate dose of morphine, sitting by the bedside and holding hands, perhaps giving them some oxygen through a small tube and allowing the angel of death to enter the room. In this regard, I am a moderately spiritual person, but I am absolutely sure that I have sat by a dying patient and felt the life force leave the body.

II

This next story is about a doctor friend, a fine surgeon with a wonderful reputation, who was beloved by his patients, and I am sure he considered himself the finest possible solution to their surgical needs. One late Sunday evening, the poor doctor died suddenly. He had three patients already hospitalized for surgery Monday morning. Yes, indeed, he was indispensable. Every one of the patients between Sunday night and Monday morning found another indispensable surgeon to operate on them and all three had their surgery as scheduled on Monday morning.

III

During my internship, I got very friendly with a father and son team of obstetrician/gynecologists. The father particularly, who was my grandfather's age, took a shine to me and allowed me to do deliveries with him and I felt very warmly toward him. His son, who was substantially my father's age, also treated me very well indeed. I mention this because not all attending physicians are inclined to treat interns very well and some of them literally abuse the staff in training. The story goes that these doctors practiced on Central Park West in a very lovely office. One entered directly from the street into a large round waiting room and the doctors' consultation rooms were to the right and left on opposite sides of this very large room. Late one night, each of the physicians was in their own offices doing paperwork when the son heard his father say, "Bob, come in here! I have a terrible pain in my chest!" The son proceeded to get up and walk across the large waiting room into his father's consultation room where he found his father slumped down on his desk dead. When the son told me this story, I was thunderstruck, extremely upset and proceeded to tell my father about it. His response was, "What a wonderful way to die." Unfortunately, my father was unable to make it to his own office, although he did, as I've said before, have seven patients in his office the night before he died.

MEMORABLE PATIENTS

I

I recall a charming young woman in the office who was wearing a tiny gold key in a chain around her neck. Rather archly, I asked her, "Where is the lock to that key?" "You should know, doctor," she said, "you've been treating it for months." I then recalled that her husband had an infected pilonidal sinus that constantly bothered him and required multiple local treatments since he utterly refused the rather extensive surgery that curing a pilonidal requires. I will not be quite so arch when I ask questions of patients in the future. Sometimes, patients are very open with these answers, but other times, of course, patients wish to be more discreet.

II

My father had a rather flighty woman in his office who required an injection. He proceeded to fill the syringe and then bulge up the skin on her upper arm to make the injection easier. She winced and pulled away from him. He said, "What's the matter? Do you bruise easily?" "No," she said, "I rape easily."

III

I'm at the old Rockaway Beach Hospital and for the day I was sent to Riis Park, it was a busy summer Sunday, and I was sent to Riis Park to be in the first aid station to try to ameliorate the zillions of minor problems that arise on a crowded beach in the summer. I treated many cuts and scrapes and crab nips and this sort of thing. Suddenly, a crew appeared carrying a young woman who was holding one knee in flexion and her kneecap was all the way over to one side of the knee. This looked extremely grotesque, she was obviously terrified and I was not too certain of the situation myself. I sent her in the ambulance to the hospital. Within twenty minutes, I got a call from my senior resident, laughing with glee over the phone. "Lou," he said, "all you had to do was straighten that knee and just tap the kneecap and it popped right back to where it belonged." Nonetheless, I am glad that I did not attempt this since I had never done or seen such a procedure before.

IV

This story concerns a wonderful, sweet woman who lived alone and out of loneliness kept three Pomeranian dogs. For those who do not know, Pomeranian are snappy, little furry lap dogs. She told my father about them only after a very long and involved situation. She had become excessively overweight and came to my father for weight loss care. He placed her on a restricted diet since he saw her as a very meticulous woman and felt that she would indeed follow such a diet. Considering her age, the only exercise she got was walking her three Pomeranian dogs and since they were small dogs, this was not major exercise. As time passed, she failed to lose any weight. My father re-enforced the diet, but she insisted that she followed the diet meticulously and could not understand why she did not lose weight. Weeks went by, and no weight loss occurred, yet she insisted that she totally adhered to the diet. Finally one day, she stopped just as she was leaving the office. (I might mention that all of the really good stuff in a medical practice is asked or discussed just as the patient is leaving the office.) Anyway, she said, "Doctor, does Schraft's Peach Ice Cream have any calories?" My father looked somewhat disturbed. "There is no Schraft's Peach Ice Cream on your diet," he said. "Oh no," she said, "my three Pomeranian dogs adore Schraft's Peach Ice Cream." Everyday I buy them a quart. But they are small dogs and they only eat a few spoonfuls each, so I finish it for them." Well, now we know why she didn't lose any weight.

V

During the 1930's, a patient appeared in my father's office complaining of a stuffy nose. He was a very interesting gentleman who had been shot during WWI and had lost the sight of one eye. When my father examined him, one nostril appeared to be blocked. After probing gently, a rather hard metallic object was encountered which was finally uneventfully removed. It turned out to be the bullet that had produced the blindness in his eye.

VI

I had a patient with high blood pressure who was very unwilling to discuss his symptoms with anybody but me. He also would frequently call at the last minute and cancel an appointment and in truth, my office staff became somewhat irritated with him. I had very warm feelings for his wife and during a visit, attempted to explain to him that my staff was irritated because of his unwillingness to divulge the reasons for changing these appointments at the last minute. He finally explained the whole thing to me. It seems that his blood pressure medicine, which was very effective at lowering his blood pressure, was unfortunately also very effective at preventing him from developing an erection. Consequently, when he or his wife became interested in the thought, he would discontinue his blood pressure medicine for a day or two so he could manage adequate sexual performance. Obviously, he knew his blood pressure would be higher and he therefore would cancel his appointment until he had gotten back on his medication. He explained to me that he really didn't wish to discuss this with my office staff and he was sorry that they didn't understand. I assured him that we would try to be flexible and informed my staff that he had a good reason for juggling his appointments and they should just accept it with good graces.

Brother Noah

When I was a small child, a fascinating patient of my father's was a very tall, broad, and powerful gentleman of color (the term of art in the 1930's) who suffered from hypertension. Brother Noah was a disciple of a charismatic preacher who called himself, Father Divine, and his disciples lived in buildings that were designated "Heavens". Brother Noah lived on the top floor of a "Heaven" in Harlem.

I might mention that female disciples where called "sisters" and male disciples were called "brothers". Interestingly, the "Heaven" that Brother Noah lived in, since I visited once with my father, was a walk-up to the fourth or fifth floor, and sort of tiring.

At all times, on a year-round basis, the disciples of Father Divine wore similar dress. The women wore white, long-sleeved, high-necked, long-skirted dresses and the men wore three piece black suits with shirts and ties. Brother Noah had an impressive gold chain across the front of his vest with a large tooth of some animal dangling from it, as well, of course, as a watch in one of the pockets. I was fascinated as a child with this gentleman and he apparently enjoyed seeing me and whenever he was in the office, he would look for me.

This is a medical story, however, and it must be noted that in the 1930's, the treatment of hypertension was weight loss, salt restriction, and basically ineffective medication mainly consisting of mild sedatives and a chemical called sodium nitrite. In any case, the years went by and Brother Noah's blood pressure was extremely difficult to control. He had no ability to change the salt in his diet since the disciples ate in a large common dining room. He had no real ability to lose weight since he was, like many of us, an excellent eater. As the years went by his blood pressure crept up and his heart got steadily larger. The standard portable blood pressure machine in those days went to 260 millimeters of mercury and eventually his systolic pressure exceeded that number.

At that point, my father switched to a wall-mounted 300-millimeter machine, but as time passed even that measurement was inadequate for Brother Noah's systolic blood pressure. Somewhere in the course of his perambulations, my father found an antique wall-mounted aneroid blood pressure machine that was calibrated to 450 millimeters, an astonishing sum, really only suitable for taking the blood pressure of Brother Noah, or a giraffe, as the case may be. In any case, that sufficed, but unfortunately, those sort of blood pressure levels cause rapid deterioration and Brother Noah developed heart failure and rather quickly died. I was quite saddened when I learned of this since I had been so attached to him. Today, of course, we have much more effective treatment for blood pressure and patients do indeed live much longer despite such illnesses.

John Hughes

In our medical unit at the old Boston City Hospital appeared one John Hughes, a strapping Irishman, florid complexion, and between each puff of his cigarette a hideous chronic cough. The cough and terrible shortness of breath had led to his admission to the hospital but that did not, in any way, decrease his interest in smoking. I should mention patients were not allowed to smoke in bed in the hospital, but there was a day hall, which also served as a lunchroom with tables and chairs. In this room there were ashtrays on every table and patients commonly went there to smoke. In nice weather they might also go outdoors since the hospital buildings were surrounded by some greenery. In any case, Mr. Hughes appeared on our unit and his chest x-ray alone basically made the diagnosis. He had far advanced multi-nodular lung cancer. Conveniently for us and for him, he also had a metastatic lymph node in his neck, which was readily biopsied to confirm the diagnosis and, indeed, the hopelessness of his case in those days. Although he was offered oxygen he rarely used it, preferring to stay upright sleeping, in fact, in a chair in his room. As time passed he became more and more short of breath but, nonetheless, was constantly smoking. His situation deteriorated to the point where he really did not sleep at night and spent most of the night sitting up in a chair in the day hall, elbows on the table, ashtray in front of him. He was found dead and cold in that position one morning still sitting in the chair, elbows on the table, head bowed, and the cigarette burnt out in the ashtray.

Mae Meyer

This was a darling, elderly woman who had been my patient for several years because of unpleasant short runs of very fast heartbeat, which distressed her greatly. Examination had disclosed a mitral valve stenosis, and, in those days, one was not rushing to operate on these patients. As time passed, the runs got worse and worse until she developed actual episodes of totally chaotic heartbeats, a condition called rapid atrial fibrillation. This was not only disturbing to her, but also made her quite ill and something had to be done. I admitted her to the hospital and after appropriate premedication got out the paddles, which by now everybody has seen on television, and proceeded to jolt her heart with a shock. This converted her immediately to a regular slow heartbeat. I decided to add a little bit of a drug called Digitalis and sent her on her way. She called several months later complaining again of the chaotic heartbeat and the situation was repeated. At the time, there were no drugs readily available that worked to keep her heartbeat regular. There are many drugs, of course, today that have been developed to do this, but at that time there were none that were effective. Consequently, periodically I would get a frantic phone call that her chaotic heartbeat was making her very ill. I would meet her at the hospital, usually in the Emergency Room, quickly sedate her, apply the paddles, and shock her heart .She would go back to regular rhythm, and I would send her home. The situation got to the point where the Emergency Room in the hospital would be expecting the two of us, and if she got there first she would be all set up with the machine waiting for me to shock her heart. What amazed me is that it always worked and lasted for some weeks to some months but, again, she always ended up back in rapid distressing atrial fibrillation. As the years went by, her heart did become weaker and weaker, and I attempted to sell her on valvular surgery but, by that time, she had read enough horror stories and decided she would just accept the heart shocks as needed. I did not see this as the best solution but was unable to persuade her otherwise. Eventually, we were unable to convert her rhythm and she expired.

PATERNALISM

As I have mentioned previously, cancer was seen as an unacceptable diagnosis and in the paternalistic days, thirty to forty years ago, it was not unusual that patients were never told that they had a cancer. The family, at some point, would be told, but this information was frequently kept from patients throughout their lives. A particular situation occurred with my own mother, who developed bowel cancer and in the course of five years underwent four operations. Nonetheless, married to a physician, the mother of two physicians, no one told her she had cancer. Of course, she never particularly asked. One day we were sitting around a coffee table with members of the family. In those days a sweetener called Sucaryl was a non-caloric sweetener that was often used. My sister-in-law mentioned casually, "You know," she said, "they say that could cause cancer." My mother, stirring her tea, smiled casually and said, "I don't have to worry."

A patient came to my father's office complaining of a strange lump on his foot. He proceeded to remove his shoe and sock to exhibit a nice clean foot and it did indeed have a very strange lump protruding from the top of the foot. My father said to him, "Let's see the other foot." The patient said, "Oh, the other foot is fine. It doesn't have the lump." My father said, "I know, but I would like to compare the two." The patient was quite reluctant, but finally, slowly removed the other shoe and sock to reveal a hideously dirty foot. My father said curiously, "Why did you wash only one foot." The patient said, "I didn't know you were going to look at the other foot."

One day my father got into a conversation with a patient who owned a bar & grill. He reminisced about the days when bars used to put out a free lunch, so-called, with salty hard-boiled eggs, salty pickles, salty meat, salty relishes and a lot of mustard. My father said that he believed that this was all done to make the people in the bar thirsty, to which the bar owner replied, "You don't have to, they come in thirsty."

OBESITY

For many years I took care of a very pleasant and intelligent young woman—she eventually became a lawyer—who was grotesquely over-weight. Although we had discussed the dieting situation many times, she never showed any real interest. At one point, she even went for a stomach stapling against my best wishes, which lasted for perhaps two months, and then she managed to gain weight again. Her mother, during an office visit, told me an interesting story. One night, while asleep, she heard rustling downstairs in her house, which awakened her. The mother was an astonishingly bold European-born woman, who kept a baseball bat in her closet. She got up and took the baseball bat and went downstairs to investigate the noise. She found her obese daughter in the kitchen stuffing handfuls of uncooked spaghetti right out of the box and into her mouth. Although this was the first time the mother had ever seen this behavior, she had seen so much grotesque overeating by her daughter, that she decided to say nothing and went quietly back to bed. The next morning, neither of them spoke about the incident again. Several years later, the daughter decided, on her own, to change her life and went on an honest to goodness long-term diet. The next time I saw her, she had lost 140 pounds and I literally did not recognize her. She did, however, get married and truly did change her life.

TATTOOS

During my medical career, I have seen many tattoos, but two in particular stick in my mind. Both of them date back to my days as a resident. One tattoo was a young woman who had tattooed on the inside of her right thigh, "pay as" and on the inside of her left thigh, "you enter". Interestingly, she was not anxious to show this to the house staff and had to be persuaded to exhibit her tattoos.

The other one was a middle-aged man who had been a Seabee. The Seabees were construction battalions during WWII and were felt to be pretty tough guys. The navy had a Seabee training base near Gulfport, Mississippi. In town, a local bar had a sign (sadly), "Niggers, dogs, and sailors keep out". One afternoon a group of Seabees entered, picked up the entire thirty foot long bar and carried it through the front window and out into the street. When the town police officer arrived, they turned over the patrol car with him in it. It took the Shore Patrol to restore order!

Anyhow, this man had the tattoo of a little face on the head of his penis with the meatus representing the mouth. He was very proud of this tattoo and showed it to anybody who wanted to ask. But when asked why he had it, the truth was he had no ready explanation. However, he insisted that it really didn't hurt to get tattooed in such a location.

MORE MEMORABLE PATIENTS

In the course of a medical lifetime, there are patients who for one reason or another stick in one's mind. Sometimes they are the patients that one fails to cure and the next doctor becomes the great diagnostician. Sometimes they're the patients that just have such unique viewpoints in life that they are memorable. Sometimes they are exasperating, challenging, critical and yet a lot of fun to care for. I will describe a few.

I had never seen him before. He was the brother of a long time patient and came from an extended family, but he had not been in my office, nor had I ever spoken to him. He had called urgently requesting an appointment. I was alone in the office doing paperwork. He came over within ten minutes, shook hands, sat down across from my desk and said nothing. He still said nothing. His face seemed very composed to me. Finally, I asked, "What can I do for you?" He paused and then finally blurted out, "I'm afraid I'm going to kill myself." This was a new experience for me and almost curiously, I said, "How do you plan to do that?" Wordlessly, he reached into his pocket, took out a pistol and put it on the desk in front of him. Equally wordlessly, I reached quickly across the desk, took the pistol and put it on my side of the desk in the lowest drawer. He appeared relieved. I suggested that we would call a psychiatrist together and set him up with an immediate appointment. Much to my relief, he agreed. A rapid appointment was quickly arranged. He left, still relieved. I called his brother and said, "Please come over and pick up this gun." His brother appeared within a few minutes and I was happy to get rid of the gun, which the brother told me was fully loaded.

Beryl

Beryl was a young married woman with several children and an adoring husband. Following one delivery she had the misfortune to have a pulmonary embolus, a serious blood clot in the lung, and was quite ill for several weeks. Obviously, she remembered this and periodically, when life became too challenging for her, she would develop the symptoms of an acute pulmonary embolus. The first few frantic house calls led to hospitalization and a lot of negative findings. As time passed, I became aware that this was an unconscious form of malingering. I became less and less impressed so the next house call, she not only complained bitterly of chest pain and shortness of breath, but her lips and fingernails were blue. However a wet Kleenex washed off the blue. She had apparently painted her lips and fingernails with blue watercolor from her children's paint set. Eventually, her complaints impressed me so little that I began to take no notice of them, and would make a house call hours and hours after her frantic emergency calls, convinced that there was nothing much the matter with her. I shortly realized that this was a grossly unfair attitude to have toward her and told her that it was time she found another doctor. I subsequently learned that some months later she had an acute abdominal episode that turned out to be a very real episode of internal bleeding from an ectopic (tubal) pregnancy. I was extremely fortunate that I had not continued to care for her because I might well have ignored this complaint also.

Bridget

Standing quietly at the foot of the bed, her heart murmur was clearly audible without a stethoscope. This was in a ward at the old Boston City Hospital, which was rarely quiet. The patient was a sweet elderly

Irish woman with a delicious brogue, which I will have to leave to the reader's imagination.

The house staff was fascinated with her and often two or three of us would be at her bedside listening to her heart. At one point, she started to laugh and told us the following story:

When I was born, the doctor told my father the baby would not live and the doctor died. When I started school, the school doctor told me that I could not take part in school recess and would have to sit quietly in the classroom and he died. When I wanted to get married, the doctor told my intended that I would never survive having children and he died. The midwife was so frightened that she demanded that a doctor come to my delivery and everything was fine. The doctor said I should never get pregnant again it might kill me. I had three more children and then the doctor died. In fact, I have a whole graveyard full of doctors who said my heart was so bad I was going to die!

Theresa

Theresa was the youngest child of a large family and remained home living with her widowed mother. During World War II, with 10 million men in uniform, women were recruited to fill all kinds of jobs ordinarily performed by men. Theresa, as a youngish woman, took a job with an aircraft manufacturing company on Long Island and was trained as a riveter. She had always been the sort of person who wanted things done correctly and, since she knew she was riveting the structure of an airplane that would be piloted by Americans, she was a totally error-free riveter. As time passed, she became an instructor in riveting for other employees and led a team of aircraft assemblers. When the war ended many women left these sorts of jobs, but Theresa just continued to do it.

I first met her in the 1970's, when she appeared complaining of headaches. At that point she weighed 200 lbs. and that matched her blood pressure exactly. Blood pressure lowering medication was helpful but I explained to Theresa that weight loss would also be a very significant factor in her long term health. I was also curious how a woman who weighed that much could squirm around inside the fuselage of airplanes under construction since she had told me that her job was a riveter. What she said to me was that her team did not let her do those jobs anymore. Seeing her as a disciplined person I gave her the world's simplest diet. I told her she could eat everything she had always eaten but, in every case, for everything she ate or drank she would devour exactly half as much. This simplistic scheme works fine except that, essentially, no one is able to keep it up for very long. Theresa came back in a month 4 lbs. lighter. And every month she came back lighter. As time passed I was able to reduce and even eliminate much of her blood pressure medication. She eventually lost 60 lbs. and went back basically to her weight when she had first started working some 30 years before. In the years that followed she eventually retired but never again gained back the weight and had totally changed her eating habits. I might mention, she is the only patient I ever saw who was actually able on that diet to completely control her weight for the long term.

Lottie

Lottie was dying of advanced ovarian cancer. It had spread to her lungs and she had been placed on a ventilator, which was keeping her alive. She communicated by writing on a pad. She wrote, "Take me off the machine." I told her she would die. "I know," she wrote. I kept up the dialogue and brought in the nurse as a witness. She kept insisting. By the time the awkward dialogue was finished, the nurse and I were both crying. The family visited, chose to leave, the switch was thrown and she stopped breathing. Morphine eased the transition and her life spirit left the room.

Ernie

Ernie was the father of one of my laboratory technicians early on in my practice. She brought him to me complaining bitterly of a backache of some month's duration. I might mention that physicians tend to remember their triumphs and forget their failures and this, I am sure, is why Ernie's case has stuck in my mind.

In any case, the physical examination disclosed many mildly enlarged abnormal lymph glands in his neck and under his arms, but no obvious problem with his back. I arranged hospitalization and in the course of the routine x-rays on admission, it was obvious that one of the bones of his spine was being eaten away probably by a malignancy. At this point the surgeon removed one of the enlarged lymph glands and under the microscope a diagnosis of what was then called "reticulum cell sarcoma" was developed. This illness, a relatively slow-growing lymphoid malignancy, was uniformly fatal in those days. Today, it is still sometimes fatal and is now called "non-Hodgkin's lymphoma". In any case, since it was a lymphoid illness, which ordinarily responds well to x-rays, we arranged to get a dozen or so x-ray treatments to his low back. This rather quickly relieved the back pain. However, we were still stuck with this essentially untreatable malignant disorder. In the course of some idle conversation with a colleague, I learned that the National Institutes of Health was doing a research project on reticulum cell sarcomas and promptly dictated a long summary of his record and, along with his biopsy slides and x-ray report, sent it off to Maryland. I received a very pleasant letter within a few days thanking me for the referral but informing me that they only were willing to accept untreated patients into their research protocol. I then started a long telephone journey to explain that the only treatment this unfortunate man had had was local x-ray treatment to the collapsed vertebrae in his spine to relieve his pain and prevent probable paraplegia and that, surely, this should not eliminate him from a potentially curative research project since the illness was so uniformly fatal. Via telephone I worked my way up the bureaucratic channel at the National Institutes of Health and finally reached a sympathetic ear with the help of a United States senator and the patient was, indeed, admitted to the research project. The family then basically moved to

Maryland to be near him during the weeks and weeks of his acute care followed by many, many months of repeated follow-up visits.

The research drugs with which he was treated were 100% successful and he was cured. I subsequently learned that this 4-drug combination therapy with the acronym "CHOP" became the standard treatment for this disease and, although not always successful, is one of the recommended treatments even to this day.

Since his daughter was a laboratory technician she was aware of the amount of effort and persuasion it took to get him accepted into this protocol. The family, I must say, was extremely grateful. In over 40 years this is really the only patient I have ever gotten the National Institutes of Health to be willing to treat.

Eli

Eli, sad to say, was not a success, but thinking about Ernie's back problem reminded me of poor Eli. Eli was the boss of a former girlfriend and, again, early in my practice she referred him to me. He had been suffering for years with a chronic backache and had had no relief from various practitioners, as well as no specific diagnosis.

When I saw him in my office he had apparently given up on doctors and had not even been seen in almost a year. On the most cursory examination it was obvious that he had a severe deformity of the spine, which could only represent intrinsic spine disease. X-ray again confirmed severe deterioration of the spine. Further study disclosed an incurable abdominal malignancy that had spread into the back and Eli, despite the treatments of the day, made a progressive downhill course and a fatal outcome ensued.

Eli's case illustrates the principle that it is always the last doctor who has the easiest time making the diagnosis in a chronic progressive illness. In Eli's specific case, after a couple of years of trying multiple doctors and not getting satisfaction, he basically gave up and saw no one for a year, just continuing to live with his back pain. The result was that when he walked into my office the obvious pathology in his back would have been impossible to miss and a simple x-ray basically made the significant diagnosis. It's one of the reasons that I tell patients with difficult problems not to abandon the quest for a diagnosis and proper treatment. Not every ailment in medicine has an easy-to-find solution.

Pat

Pat was a young woman who constantly had large nasty boils. Some of them became so severe and diffuse that she required hospitalization for intravenous antibiotics. What was astonishing is that despite adequate treatment, the boils would not only become worse, but new boils would appear. This was explained one day when a nurse caught her sticking a needle into herself. When the nurse looked more carefully, it developed that the needle had been dipped in her own stool. The mystery of the terrible infections was solved and Pat was referred for the psychiatric care she so sorely needed. Interestingly, Pat always impressed me because despite the intravenous running, she would be able to take a shower, get a haircut and travel the hospital, pushing the intravenous apparatus on a wheeled stand. At the time, it seemed almost acrobatic to me. I was a very young doctor. I have subsequently learned that you can do almost anything you want to do and maintain an intravenous.

Harry

For fifteen years, Harry suffered from a recurrent duodenal ulcer. This was in the years before our knowledge that ulcer was an infectious disease caused by a bacterium and at that time it was believed that ulcer was caused by hyper-acidity and stress and smoking. Harry did not stop smoking, he continued to be stressed and despite the best medications of the day, he continued to have recurrent episodes of his ulcer, until he finally developed so much stomach scarring that his stomach did not empty properly. At that point, I referred him for the surgical treatment, which involved cutting the nerves to the stomach and restructuring the outlet of the stomach so that it was no longer blocked. Harry had the surgery uneventfully, had none of the complications of this procedure and had complete and total relief of all his symptoms. He came back to my office about a month after surgery, furious with me, only to tell me that I had made him suffer for fifteen years when this operation would have cured him and that he and has family never wanted me to care for them again. Today, we have learned that a good course of the proper antibiotics will cure the vast majority of ulcers.

Mrs. Harry

The first member from Harry's family to call my office was Harry's wife who called for a routine check-up. When she appeared, she had no particular complaints and I proceeded, after history taking, to examine her. Medical students are taught before they examine the patient's heart with a stethoscope to palpate the patient's chest and find the point of maximal impulse of the heart's beat on the chest wall. But like many other experienced physicians, I skipped that stage and went directly to listening to the heart with a stethoscope. The tones of the heart out near the apex under her left breast were rather distant, which prompted me to move the stethoscope around and much to my surprise as I moved the stethoscope towards the center of her chest, the heart tones became much louder. I then proceeded to move slightly to the right and "eureka", the tones became louder still. At this point, I searched for the PMI and found it to be beneath her right breast. This nice lady was one of those extremely rare anomalies in which her entire body was a mirror image of the usual person. Her heart was on the right, her appendix was on the left, her liver was more on the left than the right and so forth. She was perfectly healthy but this constituted her "doctor competency test". Since I had found the point of maximal impulse on the right, I looked at her and said, "Do you know?" And she said, "Yes." It was then obvious to me that I had passed the test and at that point the entire family became my patients until the episode I have told about in the previous chapter.

Roz

Roz's husband was going blind. Roz had asthma. She deteriorated to the point where she had to be hospitalized and I put her in the local community hospital. Despite my best efforts, her condition deteriorated rather than improving with treatment. This was a little hard to understand. After a week or so with steady deterioration in her condition, I realized that she needed tertiary care and I arranged her transfer to the university teaching hospital where I had privileges. In the Intensive Care Unit, despite everybody's best efforts, including a pulmonary consultant, Roz continued to deteriorate and eventually ended up on a ventilator barely maintaining herself. In those days, intubation, the tube passing through the mouth, through the larynx, into the trachea leading to the lungs, was not too well understood, and the ventilating machines that were used at the time were much less sophisticated than the apparatus that is available today. I got a call at about 3:30 in the morning from a house officer that despite their best efforts, her blood pressure was falling and she appeared to be slipping away. I got dressed and went to the hospital. Standing at the foot of the bed, the patient appeared to be in extremis. I did not understand completely what was happening, but had the feeling something was wrong with the breathing apparatus. I was assured by the technicians that things were working properly, but I did not feel comfortable. I called anesthesia, in those days, and even today perhaps, anesthesia is the specialty of medicine that best understand the mechanics and physics of breathing machines. The anesthetist responded, also stood at the foot of the bed, said "You're overdriving her," turned the dial down by half on the volume of the respirator and within three minutes the patient looked vastly better, her blood pressure came up, she proceeded to get off the machine, recover and go home. I occasionally drive by her house and always feel good about getting out of bed that night.

Jean

In the course of one of Jean's routine visits I found a rather jolting breast abnormality. She had an area of breast skin that was edematous and pebbled (the classical textbook description is "*peau d'orange*"). Beneath this area was a thickening nodularity within the substance of the breast and, most alarming, in the armpit on that side was a walnut-sized very firm and granular-feeling lymph node. I was totally convinced that this represented a fairly advanced breast cancer. When I checked my record it turned out that Jean had not been in the office for almost three years and had not had mammograms in almost five. I informed her then and there that I was concerned that this was a quote "early cancer" and that I wanted to get a diagnosis as rapidly as possible so we could arrange appropriate treatment and that I wished to refer her to a surgeon within the next day or two. Jean looked quite worried but responded that she would have to think about this because the news was very upsetting to her and she would get back to me. When a week passed I called her and she informed me that she was still thinking about it. Her daughter was a Registered Nurse and I called the daughter, explained the situation and begged her to try to convince her mother to seek appropriate care. She informed me, and I'm afraid I realized immediately she was correct, that she had no ability to persuade her mother to do anything that she didn't want to do. In a telephone conversation a few weeks later Jean assured me that she would take care of it and that I "should not worry about it".

Many months passed. Jean burned her foot in an accident in her kitchen and called one afternoon asking to be seen. The foot was a nasty blistered burn but the treatment was quite routine and, after local treatment and a bandage, I said to her that I would like to see the breast again. On re-examination this, what I felt to be a cancerous breast, was utterly and entirely normal and the mammogram, which she willingly obtained, was also entirely normal. I do not know whether what I was seeing was my own misdiagnosis, or one of those so-called exceptionally rare spontaneous regressions of a cancer. I have no explanation for this to this day.

Approximately one year after this visit, I bumped into Jean's husband on the street and kind of idly said that I haven't seen much of his family lately. He replied that Jean felt that I had made her unduly anxious over an obviously insignificant matter concerning her breast, and that she decided to seek care with another physician.

SEX

In the course of practicing medicine, one might learn a lot about the variations in normal sexual activity. One of those that struck me was a darling young couple that came in shortly after I started practice and upon taking a sexual history, they each independently assured me that they engaged in sex two or three times a year and both expressed complete satisfaction with that situation. I did my best not to look astonished.

Under the same topic, I recall vividly a darling Irish woman who was married to man who weighted over 300 pounds. After she got to feel comfortable with me, she informed me that sex was extremely uncomfortable because he would crush her during intercourse. I suggested rather casually to her that she could be on top. A visible light bulb glowed in the air over her head as she digested this information and left the office. The next afternoon, the husband, slightly inebriated, appeared in my office to beat me up because I had interfered in his sex life and poisoned his wife's mind. I managed to talk him out of it although I never saw either of the again.

GRANDPA HARRY

Speaking about drunkenness reminds me that the most abused drug in our society by far is alcohol, and it often colors the doctor-patient relationship in so many peculiar ways. This was particularly a problem in my emergency room days but first I would like to tell you an old story from my grandfather, Harry, who was a pharmacist in the South Bronx.

In those really old days, beer was delivered to taverns only in kegs, and the kegs were tapped and served out of spigots behind the bar. People who wanted beer at home would have to bring a container to the bar, usually in those days called a tavern, and have it filled. This container was a round lidded tin with a handle and was colloquially called a growler. People would go into the saloon and order, "please fill my growler". Interestingly, even small children were sent with this covered tin down the street to get daddy or mommy a growler of beer, which was, by the way, approximately a quart.

The story goes that a very nice woman, who today we would call an enabler, used to go and get the beer for her alcohol-abusing husband. On the way home, however, with the growler full of beer, she would stop in my grandfather's drug store and have him add a couple of teaspoons of ipecac to the beer. She would then put the lid back on and deliver it to her happy husband. My grandfather's store was also a neighborhood meeting place and her husband would also come in curiously, not in any way blaming my grandfather, but just curiously. He never quite understood how when he drank in the tavern the beer sat in his stomach very comfortably but when he drank at home somehow the beer always unsettled his stomach. My grandfather, of course, did not enlighten him.

Among the more difficult emergency room cases were people who appeared drunk and injured. It is difficult enough to evaluate injuries in a cooperative patient but an uncooperative, sometimes aggressive, drunk really made everybody's life extremely difficult. Sadly, that situation persists to this day and the concerns that emergency room staff have dealing with drunken patients is one of the hazards of emergency life. Of course today emergency rooms also have the hazard of knives and guns as well as angry patients to add to their level of concern.

MEMORABLE PHYSICIANS

Emanuel Applebaum

In the course of medical education, training and practice, every doctor comes across memorable physicians and particularly during residency, there are senior staff that have very profound influences upon young doctors. I remember particularly Dr. Applebaum, known fondly as "the Apple" (not to his face of course) who was an expert in meningitis. I had occasion as a resident to treat three patients who we thought had tuberculosis meningitis (one turned out to have something else) and Dr. Applebaum's counsel was of inestimable importance and will always be with me.

Harvey Cushing

I have often felt that the greats of medicine were somehow greater 50 or 75 years ago then the so-called greats of medicine are today. I am uncertain if this is true, but it does appear that there is no real parallel today to physicians like Sir William Osler, for example. During his medical school days my father had occasion to be trained by the literally world-famous brain surgeon, Dr. Harvey Cushing. In fact, when I was a small child my father had occasion to send a contemporary of mine to Boston to Dr. Cushing, who was able to remove a frightening brain tumor and that young man, who is no longer young, of course, is still alive as I write this. Dr. Cushing had a world-famous reputation, apparently fully deserved, and is still remembered to this day.

Elliot Joslin

The diabetic guru in my father's day was Dr. Elliot Joslin who, in many ways, was seen as the father of diabetic control. I recall when my father first developed insulin dependent diabetes. He was under 50 at the time, He made a pilgrimage to Dr. Joslin, whose standard treatment involved meticulous diabetic control. It should be pointed out that meticulous diabetic control is very much acceptable today, but there was a period some 30 or 40 years ago when there were eminent physicians who felt that meticulous diabetic control was of no real value. One of the difficulties years ago was that blood sugars involved a complicated laboratory test, while the urine was readily available and somewhat simpler to test. Consequently, Dr. Joslin's patients were busy testing every urine all day and sometimes all night, and I can recall my father constantly testing urine and juggling his insulin syringe. Considering the fact that my father survived some 30 more years with his illness, it may be that meticulous control for him at least was a big plus. Unfortunately, basing meticulous control on urine has inevitable failures built in and my father had multiple episodes of insulin shock as a result of driving his blood sugar down too low with excessive amounts of insulin. He never in his life sustained a diabetic coma, so this might well be seen as a giant success.

A.A. Berg

While training at Mount Sinai Hospital, my father had occasion to be impressed with two of the surgeons on the Mount Sinai staff. A.A. Berg was generally felt to be the best abdominal surgeon in New York City at the time, and for years after he opened his office my father referred patients to him. Dr. Berg was notorious for being willing to operate on anybody no matter how seriously ill and, sometimes astonishingly, he could repair their damage and bring them through the surgery. Today, as we know, surgeons are sometimes afraid to tackle patients that are so seriously ill it appears they might die on the operating table, since these cases are often held against the surgeon trying to do his best under difficult to impossible circumstances. Dr. Berg was a very meticulous person, very demanding of his team, but notoriously he was also adored by the members of his team.

Alexis Vladimir Moskowitz

Another fascinating surgeon at Mount Sinai Hospital in my father's day was a gentleman with the above flowery name. Dr. Moskowitz, also a very busy surgeon, was practicing, of course, in the days before antibiotics. Consequently, post-operative infections did occur and the treatment required was strictly limited. One could re-operate on the patient, a very difficult procedure. One could wait until the infection cleared or localized and then drain any pus; or one could use hot compresses on the inflamed area attempting to bring the infection to the surface and drain it. Dr. Moskowitz was a great advocate of hot wet poultice dressings to the point that behind his back the house staff and the nursing staff called him "Vet Dressing Moskovitz".

Sam Bulowa

A quiet toiler in the vineyard of medicine in the 1930's was Dr. Sam Bulowa, a great social friend of my parents and, in his own way, an unsung hero. To understand Dr. Bulowa's magic I will have to review pneumococcal lobar pneumonia, the common serious lobar pneumonia, a much purer disease in the old days than it is today. The pneumococcus that causes the pneumonia is protected by a thick mucousy capsule that allows the germ to spread quickly and smoothly through the tissue of the lungs. However, different strains of the pneumococcus had different levels of virulence against humans. This virulence could be predicted by testing the sugary chemicals in the capsule of the pneumococcus germ and dozens of different types of capsular sugary materials were identified and classified. Dr. Bulowa embarked on a program to manufacture curative anti-serum against these virulent pneumococci, developing the infections in rabbits and purifying the rabbits blood serum, containing the antibodies to these capsules. This was an enormous job because of the many different types of pneumococcus capsules as well as relatively small amounts of sera that could be obtained and purified from one rabbit. Dr. Bulowa ended up with innumerable rabbits and an enormous amount of work, but eventually developed a fine system for producing therapeutic amounts of rabbit anti-serum against pneumococcal types. When a patient appeared with pneumococcal lobar pneumonia a specimen of his sputum could reveal the organism, which could then be typed, and the patient could be injected with the proper rabbit-based anti-sera. The treatment was, indeed, very effective. Unfortunately for Dr. Bulowa, just about the time he had completed this Herculean labor, taking years and years, the magic drug called sulfanilamide, followed not too long after by penicillin, completely rendered the need to type pneumococci moot. The fact was that when these drugs first appeared all pneumococci responded vigorously and quickly to these antibiotics, and far fewer patients died of these diseases.

David Scherf

When I was a senior resident at Metropolitan Hospital (in those days it was on Welfare Island), Dr. David Scherf, an enormously thoughtful and dignified gentleman of the old school, was my attending for many months at Metropolitan Hospital. I might mention that in those days a physician of the old school basically had gotten some of his training in Vienna. My own uncle, my father's brother, spent a year in Vienna to get advanced training in pulmonary medicine, and in those days it was felt that Vienna was the medical Mecca of the world. In any case, Dr. Scherf was enormously helpful in my training and I respected him tremendously.

A case that still sticks in my mind was a patient in very advanced heart failure with an enormous swollen and very tender liver. After trying all of the medications of the day with very little effect Dr. Scherf recommended we get some leeches, yes, I said leeches, and place them on his abdomen over this enormous swollen tender liver. I must say this did not make a great deal if sense to us but we went to the lower East Side, procured some leeches (they were available in those days in drug stores mainly for treating black eyes), and put three or four of them on the patient's skin where they promptly dug in and engorged themselves with blood. Amazingly the patient did indeed get some relief of his pain from his swollen liver, although his liver by all physical findings continued to be just about as swollen.

Today I wonder if the spectacle of the senior attending pontificating on this matter, followed by the application of the leeches, represented a psychological treatment of the patient as much as a medical treatment.

Lynn J. Boyd

Dr. Boyd was the Chief most of the time when I was at Metropolitan Hospital as a house officer. He was an imposing gentleman who was quite deaf and he wore a large amplifier hearing aid on a cord around his neck with a wire going to an earphone on his ear. Frequently the thing whistled mercilessly, but sometimes when he was very anxious to hear what was being said he would tilt the microphone of the big amplifier toward the source of the sound. In conferences, however, Dr. Boyd had a totally different method of dealing with sound. A case might be presented and discussion would ensue. At some point he would take the floor, and make a final firm statement that this is what he believed was wrong with this patient and this is what he believed should be done. He would then very openly reach down, shut off his amplifier, and sit back contentedly, secure that nothing anybody else said would get through to him!

While I'm on the subject of these senior physicians at Metropolitan Hospital, perhaps it's worth talking about the hospital, which was been demolished. The hospital building was originally built in the 1800's, as an insane asylum and it is mentioned, in fact described in detail, in Charles Dickens' book about his trip to America. He was particularly impressed with the central rotunda of the hospital, which had a wide circular cast iron staircase, the treads of which were 1" thick solid glass. This was such an engineering marvel in its day that there was talk of preserving that part of the hospital when it was finally torn down. I might mention that although built as an insane asylum, I treated medical patients there during my residency although the physical plant, in some ways, was more like a prison than a hospital.

Charles P. Bailey

The Chief of Cardiovascular Surgery at the Hahnemann Medical College when I attended was Dr. Charles P. Bailey, a very aggressive thoracic surgeon. We, meaning my classmates and I, believed that he was the first person to put his hand inside a beating human heart when he invented a procedure to separate fused cusps of the mitral valve, one of the four main heart valves. Dr. Bailey was a charismatic and rather demanding professor who enormously affected the aspirations of many young medical students. Over his years at Hahnemann, several students from each class would decide to become cardiovascular surgeons. At one time, as I recall, the Chiefs of that discipline at both Mount Sinai Hospital in New York and Cedars of Lebanon in California were graduates of Dr. Bailey's training program. Obviously this was a tribute, both to his expertise and his leadership in the field of cardiovascular surgery.

Philip Hensch

As a medical student, I was privileged to be able to attend Dr. Hensch's initial lecture at the Philadelphia College of Physicians auditorium. Dr. Hensch, and I am still not aware of how the idea came to him, found hideously impaired patients with rheumatoid arthritis. These were patients who were sitting in a chair for years on end, basically having everything done for them. Their joints were so seriously affected by the arthritis that they had no ability to move them.

Dr. Hensch treated these people with massive doses of cortisone and got truly magical results. He appeared at the College of Physicians to lecture on this discovery and brought with him, happily, motion pictures. I say happily because, unfortunately, Dr. Hensch had a serious speech impediment making him almost impossible to understand. At the conclusion of his lecture he then showed these unbelievable motion pictures showing people, who had been sitting for years, standing up and literally dancing for joy. As you may imagine, the audience of physicians of all ages gave him a standing ovation at the time. I can remember to this day a feeling that I had attended something truly historical and exhilarating.

Today, of course, we have learned with some sadness that although cortisone can be, indeed, a miracle drug it also has debilitating side effects, which severely limit its value in many circumstances. Sadly, this situation applies to many other advances in medicine, which are touted as true miracles when first announced, and, as the test of time ensues we find that the miracles have feet of clay. With rare exceptions, medical advances are made in a plodding fashion rather than in these exhilarating bursts of magic.

Louis B. Pearlman

Dr. Pearlman was a great colleague and personal friend of my father's. His specialty was ear, nose, and throat treatment. In those days, although obviously there could be other procedures, the standard doctor procedure for an enormous percentage of young children was a tonsillectomy and adenoidectomy. It was firmly believed that any child who developed sore throats, irritated ears, snoring, or many other nondescript symptoms would benefit from the removal of the tonsils and the adenoids. The tonsils were readily removed with a basket-shaped knife that simultaneously sliced off the tonsil and caught it in the basket. Another simple method was using a wire snare that could guillotine off the tonsil but this did not hold the tonsil and could result in serious complications. Adenoids were always removed with the basket rather than a snare since adenoid removal in those days was a totally blind operation. I might mention removal is not really the correct word. Routinely, a small portion of the tonsil was left in the throat. Often a goodly portion of the adenoid, since it was a blind operation, would also be left behind. Children were sold this procedure by being told that after the operation they could have all the ice cream they wanted which was true but, as you can imagine, they were none too happy and did not really enjoy ice cream for several days. The procedure, by the way, was performed in Dr. Pearlman's office with my father doing anesthesia. I attended these sessions many times and a goodly dozen children would be done in one morning, one right after the other, with the nurse very busy boiling, yes I said boiling, the various instruments. The pressure steam sterilization using an autoclave was not utilized in those days in private offices. I am not even sure if it was available in the 1920's in hospitals. In any case, the children would be lined up in the waiting room and zipped in and put to sleep, usually with ether, which is not a very pleasant anesthetic. The procedure would be done lickety-split and they would be kept long enough to see that bleeding was not a problem and then sent home. There were no facilities in Dr. Pearlman's office for anybody staying over night, so that all bleeding had to be controlled before evening. I might mention that Dr. Pearlman's office was in a rather nice apartment house on 93rd Street in Manhattan. The building is famous because it was the front set for the movie, "The House on 92nd Street", and the front of the building in "The House of 92nd Street" is indeed Dr. Pearlman's office even though it was on 93rd Street.

Despite the years of our father performing anesthesia for Dr. Pearlman during these tonsillectomies, I should mention that both I and my brothers have our tonsils and our adenoids to this day. A case of "do as I say, not as I do"?

Al Angrist

Dr. Angrist, who was my chief as a pathology resident, and subsequently became the Dean of The Albert Einstein Medical College, was known as "the Chief". He was called "the Chief" to his face by some of the senior residents and other attendings. This wonderful man trained basically an entire generation of pathologists. I can remember the trial of a physician who was accused of murdering a wife, or maybe more than one wife, using various anesthetic drugs. The trial became a battle of the experts and multiple pathologists were called by the defense since biochemical findings were the basis of the charges. At some point, Dr. Angrist was a witness and he proceeded to disagree with every other pathologist who had testified. The exasperated attorney finally challenged him and said, "Are you aware that you have disagreed with every one of the pathologists who have appeared before you appeared?" Dr. Angrist thought a bit and said, "They were all my boys, I guess I didn't train them very well." Astonishingly, every other pathologist on the case had been a resident trained by Dr. Angrist.

Abraham Zingher

My uncle Abraham became an expert in laboratory medicine after he arrived in America. He became such an expert that during World War I he was in charge of all the laboratory work performed on behalf of the Army in France. Upon his return from World War I, he became the Assistant Director of the Bureau of Laboratories of the New York City Health Department, which at that time was run by Dr. William Hallock Park, a world-famous epidemiologist. I should mention that the New York City Health Department Bureau of Laboratories was the premier research medical laboratory in the country and was on a par with the Pasteur Institute in France. New York State did not have a significant laboratory and, in fact, to this day I consider the New York State Health Department primarily of value in autopsying dead crows, searching for West Nile virus. The Federal Government then also had no significant laboratory facilities.

Uncle Abe was instrumental in bringing Bela Schick, the inventor of the Schick test, to New York from Vienna. He worked with Dr. Schick to improve and standardize this test (a skin test for diphtheria) and introduced it into the New York City public schools. The medical literature of the times called the test the "Schick-Zingher reaction".

My father worked for a time as my uncle Abe's assistant and, through him, was introduced to his sister-in-law. This darling woman married my father, and, as they say, the rest is history.

CONCLUSION

It is said that nostalgia is a sign of impending senility. This book has, for me, been a wonderful experience in nostalgia—medicine the way it was—less science, more art, more humanity, an ethic of service and caring above all. I am stopping, but not because I have run out of stories. New recollections pop into my head still. They repeatedly remind me of my love for, and admiration of, my father and our mutual love of the daily practice of medicine.

0-595-22925-5

www.ingramcontent.com/pod-product-compliance
Lightning Source LLC
Chambersburg PA
CBHW030812180526
45163CB00003B/1241